Having your baby when others say no!

Having your baby when others say no!

Madeline Pecora Nugent

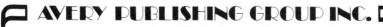

AVERY PUBLISHING GROUP INC.

Garden City Park, New York

The health and counseling procedures in this book are based upon the personal experiences, interviews, and research of the author. The publisher does not advocate any of the agencies, organizations, or individuals mentioned in this book, but believes the information presented in this work should be available to the public.

Because there is always some risk involved, the author and publisher are not responsible for any adverse effects or consequences resulting from the use of any of the suggestions in this book. Please do not use the book if you are unwilling to assume the risk. Feel free to consult a physician or other qualified health professional. It is a sign of wisdom, not cowardice, to seek a second or third opinion.

Permission Credits

p. 20. Courtesy of *Women's Touch*, March-April 1988.

p. 63. Reprinted with permission of Andre Deutsch Ltd. of London. Cardinal de Retz, *Memoirs*, from *The Harper Religious and Inspirational Quotation Companion* by Margaret Pepper (New York: Harper & Row, 1989) p. 184.

p. 104. Courtesy of Vibrant, *Genesis House News Notes*, Spring 1989.

p. 125. Courtesy of Alice Briley, "Prayer for a Small Angel," *Miraculous Medal Magazine*, December 1980.

p. 130. Courtesy of Marion Cohen, *Intensive Care #2*. Copyright 1983, Centering Corporation.

pp. 136-137. Twelve Steps reprinted with permission of Alcoholics Anonymous World Services, Inc.

p. 142. Letter to the Editor, *Newport Daily News*, Newport, Rhode Island, May 25, 1989. Reprinted with permission.

Cover Designers: Rudy Shur and Martin Hochberg
Cover Artist: Michael Apice
In-House Editor: Cynthia Eriksen
Typesetters: Straight Creek Company, Denver, Colorado

Library of Congress Cataloging-in-Publication Data

Nugent, Madeline Pecora.
    Having your baby when others say no: overcoming the fears about having your baby / Madeline Pecora Nugent.
        p.   cm.
    Includes bibliographical references and index.
    ISBN 0-89529-438-9
    1. Motherhood—United States. 2. Pregnant women—United States—Life skills guides. 3. Pregnant women—Services for—United States. 4. Childbirth—United States. I. Title.
HQ759.N84 1991
306.874'3—dc20
                                                                90-23287
                                                                CIP

Copyright © 1991 by Avery Publishing Group, Inc.

Printed in the United States of America

10 9 8 7 6 5 4 3 2 1

Contents

To all the Chrises.

Acknowledgments

Thanks to my husband, who not only supported me in my decision to write this book but who also typed portions of this manuscript. Thanks, also, to our niece who lives with us, to our children, and to friends and relatives too numerous to mention for their help and encouragement with this book. Thanks to the many professionals, including lawyers, doctors, nurses, counselors in various disciplines, and members of the clergy, for their advice and referral. Some of these people graciously read and commented on portions of this manuscript while others gave me interview time or loaned me materials. There are simply too many of these individuals to name each one. Nevertheless, I thank each.

I am especially grateful to Reverend Robert Morin and Sister Adrienne de Champlain for allowing me to utilize some of their ideas in Chapter Eight.

Thanks to Betty Yerkes, Denise Cocciolone, and LoriJo Nerad for reading the first complete draft of this book and offering suggestions. Thanks to Anna Sullivan and Dr. Robert Phillips for reading later drafts of this manuscript and sharing their insightful comments. Thanks to my editors Rudy Shur, Karen Price, Joanne Abrams, Nancy Marks Papritz, and Cynthia Eriksen for being patient as I completed this book.

To the many people who shared stories with me for this book, I am deeply grateful. The women who bore their babies are the true heroes of this effort.

Last, but most important, I am grateful to the many people who prayed for me, for this book, and for those this book will reach. I also thank Pat R., J. C., and P. R. Clete, without whom this book would never have been written.

Madeline Pecora Nugent

Preface

If you're pregnant and you want to give birth but you don't know how you're going to make it through the pregnancy and the period afterwards, this book is for you. It's also for you if you're thinking about giving birth but haven't made up your mind yet. Is it possible for you to work through your problems and have your baby? What adjustments will you have to make? How can you make them? No matter what your problems, this book will answer your questions and provide information that you probably never thought existed.

This book is not a balanced discussion of abortion. If you want information on abortion, you can find many books and articles on the topic. Those resources tell you how to *end* a pregnancy. This book tells you how to *continue* it.

If you're like most people, you're unaware of the vast network of help available. You certainly don't want to handle your pregnancy all alone, especially if you are poverty-stricken, distraught, or ashamed of your pregnancy—and you don't have to. This book provides guidelines that will help you change from a victim of your situation to a victor over it. It really is possible to bear your baby and have a future at the same time.

Several years ago, I looked for a book like this one. I had gone through two minor pregnancy crises myself. In one case, I was pregnant at a very inconvenient time; in the other, the baby was due to be born at the beginning of an extremely busy six-month interval of my life. The only book I found to help me was reassuring, yes, but it offered no specific guidelines. I was left with the feeling that my life would work out if I gave birth, but I didn't know how I was going to make that happen. However, I was fortunate. I had some idea of what to do.

At the time of my first pregnancy crisis, I had been a volunteer crisis pregnancy counselor for almost six years. Even though I was too busy with my two little children to spend time in the crisis pregnancy office, women were calling me at home. For years, I searched for a book that would give these women some solid direction and information. Most of these women had crises far worse than mine. And some had unbelievable difficulties. Yet they wanted to be strong enough emotionally to work through the problems and give their babies a chance. I could find self-help books on all sorts of other problems. Why nothing on this? During my second pregnancy crisis, my own experiences, combined with my knowledge that thousands were grappling with their own crisis pregnancies, convinced me that I had to write the book you're looking at now.

If you're like most women reading this book, you're facing more than one problem. You may even have several severe problems that make it difficult to carry your baby to term. Difficult, but not impossible. This book is designed to help you work through your problems, either by yourself or with the help of others.

Chapter One will help you define your problems and understand why you feel compelled to give birth, even though many of your emotions are pulling you in the opposite direction. If you're interested in your unborn baby's development, Appendix A will give you some idea of how your baby is developing. Appendix D will help you focus on just exactly what is bothering you about pregnancy and birth. You will probably want to discuss some of your questions with a counselor. Appendix I lists reading material that may help with specific concerns.

In Chapter Two, you'll learn how to meet your basic needs, beginning with the confirmation of your pregnancy and the concealment of it until you're ready to tell the world. And, if you don't want to tell anyone, you'll discover how to keep your pregnancy a secret. In Chapter Two, you'll learn the vital techniques of managing stress and thinking positively so that you can pinpoint your emotions and use them to define your problems. Keeping a journal will help you organize your thoughts and work toward obtaining all the necessities of pregnancy, including shelter, food, money, clothing, medical and other professional care, and a supportive, trustworthy friend. Appendix H lists many agencies that may be able to provide help, answer questions, or make referrals.

Because other people can, often unwittingly, make a pregnancy crisis even more alarming, Chapter Three explains how you can handle others. In this chapter, you will find tips on choosing a good doctor and other qualified professionals. You'll decide how, when, and if to reveal your pregnancy to your family and friends, teachers and fellow students, coworkers and bosses, and community and religious groups. An entire section contains suggestions on successfully managing your love life during pregnancy. In addition, you'll learn how to deal with rejection, social stigma, and abuse, and you'll read about particular techniques for handling an increasing problem, namely, dealing with pregnancy while in prison. Appendix F presents a list of questions to ask when assessing the influences of your lover, your career and educational goals, and others on how you deal with your pregnancy.

If either you or your baby faces health difficulties, you may want to refer to Chapter Four. With more and more people suing doctors for malpractice, doctors have become extremely cautious in treating pregnancy. They may want to caution you about all possible complications and outcomes, and attempt to influence your decisions. Chapter Four has suggestions on dealing with this type of pressure. You need to be aware of your rights and responsibilities. Appendix E has questions you should ask professionals and yourself as you choose medical options. With this information, you will be able to make better decisions based on complete information.

Chapter Four also addresses concerns about your health. The chapter discusses environmental influences, over-the-counter medications, illegal substances, birth control methods, stress, inherited defects, and other factors that can affect your developing child. You will read about the advantages and limitations of prenatal testing and of second opinions so that you can make wise decisions regarding whether to take a test and what course of action to follow if a problem is discovered.

If you're reading this book, you probably are seriously considering giving birth. But you may not know if you want to or are able to parent your baby. Even if you are married, giving birth does not automatically mean that you will be responsible for parenting. Today, more than ever before, adoption, foster care, institutional care, and legal guardianship are widely available to married and single women alike. Chapter Five explains the new trends in adoption that can help you keep in touch with your adopted children, if you so wish. It also gives some practical tips on parenting in various situations, and discusses different types of families so that you will be able to choose a parenting option wisely. Appendix G presents questions that you should ask yourself as you clarify your preferences.

Your pregnancy crisis may involve traumas that most other women will never face. These may involve pregnancy from rape, incest, prostitution, or sexual addiction. You may be unhappy with past sexual behavior, yet not know how to avoid the same behavior in the future. Or you may have emotional scars from past sexual encounters, some forced on you and others freely chosen. Chapter Six deals with all of these problems, and gives guidelines for successfully overcoming them.

Chapter Seven will help you if you face any one of several other painful situations. In rare cases, you may face death if you give birth; yet, you may want to choose this option. What arrangements must you make? Chapter Seven provides some guidance. If your pregnancy is so threatening that suicide sometimes seems like a good option, Chapter Seven tells you there is hope and shows you how to find help.

Prenatal testing may reveal that your unborn baby has special needs or is dying. Should you parent? How can you? How can you respond if you know that giving birth means saying good-bye? Chapter Seven, as well as Appendix B and Appendix G, will guide you in your decisions. Appendix C deals with helping the mentally retarded mother through her pregnancy and afterwards, and gives direction about finding help for those working with her.

Sometimes, a current pregnancy brings back painful memories of a previous abortion. You must face these emotions if you are to have the peace you need to deal with your current pregnancy. Sadly, every woman has some chance of having her pregnancy end unexpectedly in miscarriage, stillbirth, or infant death. Chapter Seven gives advice and comfort to mothers dealing with these painful situations.

No matter how overwhelming it seems, this pregnancy crisis is only a small portion of your entire life. However, it may make you realize the need for greater control over your other circumstances. For this reason, Chapter Eight offers some guidance for your future personal and, if you wish, spiritual growth. Thinking positively about yourself, seeking counseling, using self-help groups, and deepening your faith experiences are all ways to grow stronger emotionally. Chapter Eight points you in the direction of this ongoing growth.

While using this book, keep in mind a few very important points. Every pregnant woman should be under a doctor's care. While this book discusses medical problems, it does not attempt to recommend treatments for specific conditions. If you face the medical problems discussed in this book, or any other medical problems, you must seek the advice of competent physicians before making decisions regarding your pregnancy.

In the same way, if you face mental or emotional difficulties, you must seek the advice of competent professionals trained in the fields of mental health and counseling before reaching a decision. If you're making legal decisions, you should consult legal experts about applying the information in this book to your specific case. Finally, you should consult specific PREGNANCY AIDgencies or other groups for assistance with specific problems.

While this book offers much advice, it cannot address each woman's specific situation. Neither the author nor publisher shall be liable for the outcome of any pregnancy or the results of decisions made by anyone who follows the suggestions in this book.

This book and its appendices mention several agencies, organizations, individuals, and books that may help pregnant women who wish to give birth. Mention of these agencies, organizations, individuals, authors, publishers, and others does not imply that they adhere to any religious, political, or social philosophy regarding abortion or any other issue.

Keep in mind a few points when you feel frustrated during your pregnancy. Don't give up when seeking help. If one group or agency won't or can't help, look elsewhere. Help is available. This book will tell you how to get it. You *can* give birth to your baby and make wise decisions about parenting. Don't ever give up looking for help!

Above all, believe in your abilities. If you think you have very few, this book will help you discover many more. If you want to have your baby, you, like the women whose stories appear in this book, possess the courage and determination inside of you to see this pregnancy through. I believe in your strength. I believe in your creativity. Believe with me.

Madeline Pecora Nugent

Introduction

Dear Woman in Crisis,

I feel your pain, despair, confusion, and anger. It's OK to cry, to curse, and to shriek what you are feeling.

You feel frightened. Trapped. Without hope. Unable to cope. You feel that your future is being destroyed by the child within you. Your baby's future or your own? How can you decide?

You need not choose between your future and your child's. You can both have a good future. You can both live well.

You will learn, like so many other women, that the enemy is not your baby. Instead, the enemy is fear, self-doubt, anger, pride, envy, and perfectionism. *Fear* of rejection. *Self-doubt* about making decisions, following through, and persisting when life gets hard. *Anger* about this unforeseen crisis. *Pride* that makes you resist help and change. *Envy* of others' talents, time, and resources. *Perfectionism*, which believes that life should always be easy and always be planned.

Maybe you're used to being a superwoman, handling things alone and helping others. Now is the time for others to help you and your baby. Many people are willing to help you. This book will tell you where to find those people and how to help yourself. Reach out to them!

Reach up! Expand yourself and your abilities. Almost 2,000 years ago, Paul of Tarsus wrote, "There are three things that last—faith, hope, and love." Not perfection. Not planning. In faith, hope, and love, reach for a brighter tomorrow. You will have it.

Reach deep! You have a hidden strength and this book will help you find it. Things you never dreamed of are within your power. Believe in yourself.

Love yourself. You have the ability to handle this pregnancy, to make good decisions, and to give birth, even if others are telling you "no."

Believe that you will emerge from this crisis a stronger, better woman. Because you will.

Madeline Pecora Nugent

Having your baby when others say no!

Chapter One

PREGNANCY CRISIS— FIRST REACTIONS

"Patience is both virtue and victory."

—*M.P.N.*

Solving Your Problems—One at a Time

Throughout this book are examples of women who became pregnant in situations that were less than ideal. Each of these women experienced a crisis pregnancy, one in which the mother encountered some type of hardship and had to act to resolve a problem. Uncertainty about what to do plagued these mothers. Their names, and some other details, have been changed to protect their privacy. If someone you know was in a situation similar to and has the same name as somebody described in one of the stories, it is purely coincidental. Every pregnant woman's name, without exception, was changed in this manuscript. However, if you are pregnant and are reading this book to help yourself decide what to do, you may be like at least one of the very real women in these examples.

Maybe your situation is similar to fifteen-year-old Sheila's. She wanted to have her baby, but her parents insisted that she abort.

Or perhaps you are like Jo, who, when she became pregnant, was depressed, unwilling to continue her education, jobless, and homeless. Her college lover offered to pay for an abortion.

Maybe you are recently married, like Lisa and Tyrone, who were just barely making ends meet when Lisa became pregnant unexpectedly.

Maybe you are a victim of rape, like Sarah. A single woman with a physical disability, Sarah lived in a small town and became pregnant after a married acquaintance raped her.

Perhaps you are in Dora's situation. When a routine test indicated that Dora's baby was mentally retarded, both she and her husband agreed not to raise a child with special needs.

Or you may be an older mother like Mae, who married at thirty-five and decided that she was too old to be a parent. At age forty-five, she discovered that her "menopause" was actually pregnancy.

Your situation may differ from any of these. Like you, all of these women were in a crisis. And all gave birth to their babies. How did they do it?

FOUR TRAITS FOR SUCCESS

Sheila, Jo, Lisa, Sarah, Dora, and Mae had four common traits that helped them through their pregnancies. These traits can be developed in anyone, including you.

Like Yourself

Learn to like yourself! When you like yourself, you'll like your baby, too. You'll want to make plans to help you both. Sure, you have room for improvement—we all do. But you are still worthwhile. Why? Because you're you! You want to give your baby a chance. Only someone special can do that.

You can talk yourself into liking yourself. Look in a mirror and say your name. Then add, "I want to like myself. I will try to like myself. I know that I am valuable. I like myself." If you do this exercise often, you'll soon mean what you say. Think positively about yourself.

If you have difficulty liking yourself, speak to a friend, psychologist, counselor, or member of the clergy. Talk about why you don't like yourself. Ask your counselor to help you see the good inside of you. You may need to heal some wounds and get rid of guilt in order to like yourself.

Face Up to Your Crisis Pregnancy

Make sure you're pregnant, following the guidelines in Chapter Two. Denial is common in pregnancy. If you are pregnant, admit it! Once you admit to yourself that you *are* pregnant, then admit that you can't run from your situation. You can't go to a "crisis clinic" and simply end a crisis, no matter what your situation is. You have to face and work through your problems. Your pregnancy will end, with your baby's birth or otherwise. This book will help you end your crisis.

Discover the Real Problem

You see, *pregnancy is not your real problem.* The *real* problem involves the circumstances and people that make this pregnancy difficult.

For example, if you were healthy, happily married, and financially secure, with a supportive family and a healthy, planned baby and no other difficulties in your life, your pregnancy would not be a problem. You are experiencing problems because your life differs from this ideal picture. Ending your pregnancy will not change the circumstances or the people in your life. They will all exist whether you are pregnant or not.

In order to solve your problems, you have to see the "big picture." You'll either have to change the circumstances and people that are troubling you, or learn to deal with them.

Take One Knot at a Time

How will you solve your problems? The same way you untangle a mass of yarn—one knot at a time. As much as we would like to have our futures clearly mapped out, we must face each day as it comes, with the problems and surprises it brings. One problem faced, one problem solved—one problem at a time.

Before your baby is born, you have months to plan. This book will help you. Right now, why not skim through this book? Skip the parts that don't apply to you and concentrate on the ones that do. You'll get ideas on how to handle your crisis. Go back and reread the sections that apply to you.

AND NOW YOU'VE BEGUN

Believe it or not, you've begun to deal with your situation! You know you have difficulties. You know you need help. Yes, some decisions will be difficult, but you are trying to believe in your ability to make them. You're beginning to feel more confident about giving both yourself and your baby a future that will make you proud.

> *"If you can't have Life as you want it,*
> *want Life as it is."*
>
> *—M.P.N.*

Bothering With a Pregnancy

A crisis pregnancy sometimes involves feelings of guilt. It could be guilt about how you got pregnant. About the poor timing of the pregnancy. About wanting to give birth against the advice of those around you. About angering or disappointing someone. About not wanting to raise a baby. You may feel guilty enough to choose to have an abortion, even though you don't really want one.

Pregnancy itself brings depression, because rapid hormonal changes cause depression and mood shifts in every pregnant woman. Any veteran mother and/or seasoned obstetrician will tell you that even in the most well-planned and long-anticipated pregnancies, hormones wreak havoc on a woman's emotions. The result is great confusion in even the most dedicated mothers. Luckily, this passes as the pregnancy progresses. In a crisis pregnancy, the hormonal influences are especially upsetting because your crisis creates depression, too. You think nothing will work out, so why try?

Guilt and depression are states of mind, not flags signaling defeat. Yes, you have problems and have made mistakes. Who hasn't? Let go of guilt and depression. They will keep you from making good plans for your baby's future.

PEOPLE WHO CREATE GUILT AND DEPRESSION

Avoid people who are especially good at creating guilt and depression. These people might make you feel guilty either for getting pregnant or for wanting to give birth.

There are people who like to have complete control—the **planners**. They believe that life should be perfectly planned. They ignore the reality that plans sometimes go astray. If someone asks, "Was your pregnancy planned?" reply, "That's a personal question." Some people may think that you should abort a baby you didn't plan on having. You may feel that your baby deserves a birthday.

Sad sacks have the attitude that life is always most unfair to them. They will see your pregnancy only as a negative thing, a burden. Don't listen to them. Planning and help can lighten even the heaviest burden and turn your baby's birth into a wonderful experience.

Authoritarians are overpowering and manipulative, locked in a struggle for control. These people may try to badger you into giving birth to your baby. You might rebel and want to choose abortion just to prove that you can decide for yourself. Don't choose to have an abortion that you don't want in order to retaliate against authoritarians.

Fantasizers think that life should always provide happiness. "Just get an abortion and forget your pregnancy ever happened," they say. Sometimes their advice sounds tempting.

Blacklisters think that you never do anything right and that you care only about yourself. If you listen to them, you might come to believe this. "Maybe I am self-centered. I don't care about my baby, so why give birth?" But you do care. That's why you're reading this.

Sanctifiers view you as almost perfect. You're trustworthy, dependable, kind, and intelligent. Sanctifiers expect you to choose abortion so you don't disappoint or worry anyone. If you want to have your baby, an abortion may disappoint and worry you. Put yourself first for a change. Do what's best for you.

WHOSE CHOICE?

Is abortion really your free choice, or are you choosing it because you are influenced by depression, guilt, or the reactions of others? Will you choose abortion just to please someone else? Soon you'll learn how to deal with your feelings and with those of others. You'll be able to make a firm plan for your pregnancy and childbirth that others will learn to accept.

IF YOU NEVER WANTED A CHILD

Maybe you never wanted children. Now you're pregnant, and you're really confused. You don't want a child, but abortion makes you uneasy. You don't really want that either.

Do you know why you don't want children? Finding out will help you understand the emotions you must work through in order to have your baby.

Appendix D has a series of questions that will help you discover why you don't want a child. Answer these questions alone or with a trained counselor. You may be surprised at what you will learn about yourself.

What Is Your View of Children and Parenting?

Maybe you dislike or misunderstand children, or expect too much of them. Perhaps you can't visualize yourself as a parent or don't want to parent. In order to have your baby, you might need accurate information on childbearing and parenting. Perhaps you have to heal the angry, frightened child who still lives in your memory.

Upon their marriage, Rebecca and Craddock figured that they would be able to overcome their unhappy childhoods and poverty if they worked hard and remained childless. After trying unsuccessfully to end a late-in-life pregnancy, they came to love their daughter Karen and gave her many opportunities to become a teacher, lecturer, and world traveler. Karen cared for both her parents when they became terminally ill. During that time, Rebecca apologized for not being able to show her daughter more love. Yet Karen had learned love. Those who knew her said she blended compassion and humor in dealing with her students.

What Is Your View of Men and Women?

You have a certain view of men. You may feel that men will find you unattractive if you're pregnant. Or perhaps you believe that men have used pregnancy as an excuse to keep women in secondary roles. You may reject your pregnancy because you think it could be a negative influence on your love or work relationships with men.

You also have a certain view of yourself as a woman. In a way, it might be said that rejecting pregnancy is denying your biology, your womanhood. Maybe you think that being pregnant means being weak, but that's not true. Going through a pregnancy, especially a crisis pregnancy, taking charge, and making decisions may require that you be the strongest you have ever been.

Perhaps you, like fashion designer Yolanda, want to be totally free to pursue your chosen lifestyle. Like her, you may feel that a woman can find fulfillment without raising children. That's why Yolanda and her husband felt perfectly comfortable continuing their careers throughout Yolanda's two pregnancies and then making adoption plans for their two children.

In order to give birth, you need to know just how you view men and women. Are your views valid? How can you give birth and still maintain the views you hold?

What Is Your View of Change?

Being pregnant definitely means facing changes in your body, physical activities, and plans. In addition, you will try to imagine how your life will change if you parent your baby or if you make an adoption plan.

The only thing constant about life is change! Yet many people fear change. The fear of change can cripple you. You may be tempted to end your pregnancy so that you don't have to face the changes pregnancy will bring.

How do you see change—as a challenge or as a threat? What changes necessitated by your pregnancy are you dreading? Try to view change as a chance to improve yourself and expand your experience. Change can be good!

Hannah and her husband are both blind. After being told that Hannah could not get pregnant, the couple became foster parents to children with disabilities and adopted a few of them. When Hannah became pregnant, she was so afraid she'd love her adopted children less that she didn't want her baby.

After much emotional turmoil and a difficult pregnancy, Hannah gave birth to a blind, gifted daughter whose deafness disappeared without treatment. Hannah soon realized that she had enough love for all of her children—her adopted children and her newly born daughter.

ENDING A PREGNANCY

Pressure to end a pregnancy can come from others or from mixed emotions within yourself. It's tempting to "end it all" quickly, before you change your mind. But these nine months of pregnancy are less than 1 percent of the average lifetime. It is possible that you may never be pregnant again.

Sometimes ending a pregnancy might seem as simple and quick as removing a thorn. Is it? Because you are pregnant, your body feels different. Your mind knows that a new life is beginning, even if you don't like to think about it. You'll remember your trip to the abortion clinic, the procedure itself, and the sensations you feel afterwards as your body returns to its nonpregnant state. You'll also remember the obstetrician-gynecologist who gives you a follow-up exam to make sure that no problems or infections resulted from the abortion.

If you're like most post-abortal women, you'll start to notice pregnant women and babies and recall your abortion sequence. Often, ending a pregnancy leaves many memories. Sometimes, it can leave emotional scars.

If you don't really want an abortion, reaffirm your decision to have your baby. Life is not always the way we want it to be. Sometimes we have to accept life the way it is. Accepting your pregnancy is a beginning toward making your life all it can be.

Chapter Two

GETTING THROUGH
THE PREGNANCY

"First choices are often the most important ones."

—M.P.N.

Confirming, Confiding, Caring, Concealing—
the Four C's of Pregnancy Crisis

CONFIRM YOUR PREGNANCY

Some women assume that they are pregnant just because they have missed a menstrual period. Are you sure you're pregnant? You may not be! Now you have to make sure. There are several ways that you can find out if you are pregnant.

Use a Home Pregnancy Test

Most pharmacies sell home pregnancy testing kits. Call a pharmacy to make sure. If you live in a small town and are afraid of being recognized, disguise your voice or have a friend call, or choose an out-of-town pharmacy. Follow the kit's instructions carefully.

Modern pregnancy tests claim to be accurate if performed at least one day after a missed period. But, if a test indicates that you're *not* pregnant and you don't get your period, take another pregnancy test in two or three weeks just to make sure. If this test is also negative, consult your doctor. You may have a medical problem in need of treatment.

Consult a Doctor

Obstetricians, gynecologists, and general practitioners usually can perform pregnancy tests. Call a local or out-of-town doctor and make an appointment. If you must go to a hospital to have the test done, a doctor will make arrangements.

It is best to think of your doctor only as a medical caregiver. Unfortunately, many doctors are poor crisis pregnancy counselors. You may have one who is compassionate and encouraging, but if a doctor discourages you from having your baby, refer to this book for advice.

Use a PREGNANCY AIDgency

You won't find a phone book listing that reads "PREGNANCY AIDgency." This term is not the name of a specific agency, but rather is this book's general term for social service agencies that deal exclusively with women in pregnancy crises and help them give birth to their babies. Over 3,000 local PREGNANCY AIDgencies exist worldwide under different names such as Birthright, Lifeline, Helpline, and others. These names and others may be listed in your phone book. Most do free pregnancy testing and can offer you help in many other ways as well.

To locate a local office, call one of the national hotlines listed in Appendix H at the end of this book. If you get an answering machine, leave your first name and phone number or else call back when the AIDgency is open.

Family Planning Clinics—A Word of Caution

Family planning clinics and abortion clinics frequently advertise free pregnancy testing. However, these clinics make money by performing abortions and may encourage you to consider one without offering the options listed in this book. If you want to have your baby, a very caring abortion counselor will only distress and confuse you if the counselor is convinced that this pregnancy will ruin your life. No matter what you're told, you *can* give birth to your baby. This book tells you how.

Some abortion clinics advise over 85 percent of the women who test positive for pregnancy to have abortions, according to JoAnn Gaspar, a former employee of Planned Parenthood. Debra Henry, a certified medical assistant who assisted at an abortion clinic, explains. "We were told to find the [pregnant] woman's weakness and work on it. The women were never given any alternatives. They were told how much trouble it was to have a baby." Knowing this, you can decide if you want to go to an abortion clinic at all.

To research an article on abortion counseling, happily pregnant Krystal made an appointment at an abortion clinic. Her own doctor had spoken to Krystal about her four-month-old baby and had allowed her to watch the child on the ultrasound for almost an hour. The clinic counselor never mentioned the word "baby" and positioned the ultrasound screen so that Krystal could see nothing. Even though Krystal said she hadn't thought through the decision to abort, the counselor discussed no alternatives to abortion and, instead, assured Krystal that the "termination procedure" was like "having a tooth pulled." Krystal's article was published in a national magazine. Krystal gave birth to her much loved daughter.

CHOOSING A CONFIDANT

A pregnancy crisis is a frightening time to be alone. You need a friend in whom you can confide your deepest hopes and fears. But who?

Choosing the right confidant will be one of the most important decisions you will ever make. The right confidant will encourage and support you, dispelling much of your stress and tension.

You wouldn't be reading this book if you didn't want the best for yourself and your baby. The wrong kind of confidant will offer opinions without really considering what is best for you and your baby. He or she may be kind, intelligent, and well-meaning. But if this confidant is pressuring you to abort your baby, you will experience much additional stress and tension. You don't need any more of that, do you?

Finding the Right Friend

A volunteer from a PREGNANCY AIDgency should make an excellent confidant. These volunteers are trained to both help and support you. Why not give your local PREGNANCY AIDgency a call? When calling long distance, call collect so that you won't have to pay for the call. Try to visit your confidant, too.

Secret Testing in Progress

Suppose you have someone other than a PREGNANCY AIDgency volunteer in mind for your confidant. How can you tell if this person will support you?

Strike up a conversation with the person you are considering confiding in. Casually bring up pregnancy problems or abortion, focusing on something currently in the news. Or discuss someone who had a surprise pregnancy, or a book or movie with a crisis pregnancy in the plot.

How does your potential confidant respond? People may respond in the following ways.

- No matter how kind or well-meaning a person is, don't confide in someone whose remarks are very much in favor of aborting your baby. Such remarks might include, "Abortion is a legal right. It's the best choice." "I don't know why women have babies they didn't plan." "The world is too populated already." "An unplanned baby can ruin your life." "Abortion is the best way out of a bad situation."

  People have a right to these opinions. However, no matter how nice these people are, they are likely to attempt to persuade you to abort your baby.
- Consider confiding in someone who is against abortion. This person might say, "A woman can always choose adoption." "A baby should have a chance." "If women would just have faith, God would help them give birth." "A woman might have problems because of an abortion."

  If this person is kind, clear-thinking, and nonjudgmental, you may have found an excellent confidant who will stick by you through good times and bad, right up to and even after the birth.
- Many people claim that abortion should be a personal choice. "It's up to a woman to decide." "I would never have an abortion myself, but I can't stop someone else from having one." "A woman has to live with her own decision." "I don't like abortion, but if a woman thinks she needs one, it's her choice."

  A proponent of abortion who is honestly pro-choice should accept your choice to give birth and should help you to carry out that choice. However, some people who claim to be pro-choice may believe that abortion is almost always the best choice. These people may try to persuade you to believe this, too. Take care in choosing your confidant to ensure that this individual is most interested in your plans—not in a personal agenda.

This Is the One!

Keep chatting with potential confidants until you find one who seems supportive. Ask your confidant to keep your secret and invite your confidant to stand by you and to help you. If you find that you've made a poor choice, quiz others and choose again.

> *With two adolescent children, a recently born baby she hadn't planned on having, and a husband who had just gone bankrupt, Harmony got pregnant again. By confiding in a pro-life friend and keeping her pregnancy hidden until her sixth month, Harmony slowly worked through her depression and anger, and came to believe that God had a plan for her baby. Her husband got a new job, and her baby girl brought great joy to her family.*

CARE FOR YOUR BABY AND YOURSELF

Every pregnant woman needs to be under a doctor's care from the very beginning of her pregnancy. A doctor will prescribe prenatal vitamins, which will keep you and your baby healthier, and will be able to spot and treat any medical problems that arise. For your own health and that of your baby, you need to choose a doctor now.

Of course, you want a doctor who will be supportive of your decision to give birth. Not all doctors will feel this way. Chapter Three and Appendix E will tell you how to choose a supportive doctor. Refer to these sections now.

If you are embarrassed by your pregnancy, or don't want others to know about it, you may feel very uneasy about seeing a doctor. Ask a PREGNANCY AIDgency to refer you to a good doctor in a nearby area, or consult the phone book to find a doctor who does not know you. Remember, a doctor should not broadcast your pregnancy to the world, or even to your parents or partner, if you don't want others to know.

CONCEAL YOUR PREGNANCY

If you're not blessed with supportive family and friends, it's probably best to conceal your pregnancy until you have a plan for dealing with it. By waiting several months, some people who would have pressured you to abort will think that you are "too far along." By then, you'll feel more confident and at peace because you will be working out ways to give birth. You can carefully plan if, how, and when to announce your pregnancy and your pregnancy plan to others.

For now, do not mention your pregnancy to anyone who might discourage or pressure you, not even a parent or lover. Confide in your confidant and doctor only. The following suggestions will help you conceal your pregnancy.

- Act cheerful and untroubled. Practice looking happy before a mirror until you feel more comfortable. Get your rest by going to bed earlier or spending time in your bedroom. If you share a room, see if you can rest at your confidant's house. If nausea is a problem, refer to the advice given later in this chapter.
- If you engage in strenuous physical activity or have a potentially dangerous job, tell your doctor. If necessary, your doctor can exempt you from some physical activities or request safer working conditions without making your pregnancy public.
- Practice good posture. Slouching emphasizes your belly. Good posture makes your tummy recede into your waistline. Ask your doctor for some posture exercises for pregnant women, or consult a library book.
- Wear concealing clothing, not maternity clothes. Although your stomach may look fat to *you*, proper clothing can conceal the bulge from others for at least five to seven months. Fasten your jeans or skirts with pins or leave the snap and zipper open. Choose long, large, loose bulky sweaters, T-shirts, jogging suits, men's shirts, or oversized blouses. Consider elastic-waisted slacks in a larger size; billowy, oversized fashions; or suits with concealing jackets. Purchase maternity pantyhose and you needn't worry about them slipping. As you gradually switch to looser styles, people will assume you've changed your wardrobe or that you've gained a little weight.

Gayle's wardrobe of tasteful suits and loose dresses was perfect for hiding her unexpected pregnancy, especially since Gayle had beautiful posture. She wanted to parent her baby but hid her pregnancy until the eighth month, even from her other four children, the youngest a preteen. At forty-two, Gayle was campaigning for public office after recovering from an extremely malignant form of abdominal cancer. She did not want her family to pressure her to stop campaigning or to choose abortion, as her doctors, who feared the pregnancy might cause the cancer to recur or spread, were doing. Ten days after losing her bid for office, Gayle gave birth to a son whom she calls "a gift from God."

FOLLOW THE FOUR C'S

Confirm your pregnancy—then you can begin planning for your baby. Find a **confidant** to share your burden. Choose a good doctor to **care** for you and your baby. **Conceal** your pregnancy until your plans are firm. Soon your crisis will turn into cradlesong.

"A secret's a secret if only trustworthy folks know."

—*M.P.N.*

Keeping Your Pregnancy a Secret

Not every woman has to conceal her pregnancy. In many areas, unmarried moms are common and generally well accepted. Think carefully about whether you *really* need to keep your pregnancy a secret and from whom. Being truthful is always much simpler than keeping any secret.

However, you may come from a very conservative family or a very conventional area. You may be in an abusive or threatening environment. Possibly, you have a very good reason for keeping your pregnancy a secret. But can you really conceal your pregnancy and give birth to your baby? Yes, you can.

Most women who keep their pregnancies secret make adoption plans for their babies as Andrea, Kathleen, and Farrah (mentioned later in this chapter) did. Chapter Five and Appendix G will help you make an adoption plan.

MAKING A PLAN

You may want to keep your pregnancy a secret from your family and friends, but somebody will have to know. The best thing to do is to contact a PREGNANCY AIDgency to devise a safe, comfortable plan. You will probably need to consider one or all of the following in making plans to conceal your pregnancy.

Overcoming Embarrassment

If you're unmarried but embarrassed by your pregnancy, wear an inexpensive wedding band. If anyone mentions your husband, you could say, "All that guy left me is this baby. I prefer not to talk about it." This statement avoids lying, keeps people from prying, and leaves you free to date.

If a new relationship begins to get serious, tell this desirable man the complete truth. If he loves you, he should be able to accept your pregnancy. A PREGNANCY AIDgency volunteer or other counselor can help you tell him lovingly and gently.

Alibis

If you move away to give birth, you need a believable alibi for going. In your new location, a PREGNANCY AIDgency can help you get a job, continue your education, or learn a skill. You can tell those at home that you're visiting friends, taking a vacation, or caring for a relative. Or say you've been under a lot of stress (don't say why) and a doctor has ordered you to get away for a while. You could make up a unique excuse.

Andrea and Kathleen used these techniques to hide their pregnancies forever, even from their families. Andrea said she was "going on vacation" but, instead, went to a PREGNANCY AIDgency shelter home and gave birth. Kathleen went away to college and gave birth in the college town. Andrea returned home with postcards, and Kathleen with college credits, without anyone suspecting that the two had been pregnant. Wealthy, prestigious Farrah's parents would not even tell the PREGNANCY AIDgency their daughter's real name as she took an extended trip out of the country. All three of these women made adoption plans.

Other Children

If you have other children, what arrangements will you make for them? Can a friend or relative care for them if you go away? Could you have a nanny in your home? Could your children go with you? A PREGNANCY AIDgency can help you make plans.

Permanent Relocation

Some women move elsewhere permanently. Maybe you'd like to start out fresh someplace else. When you decide where, ask a PREGNANCY AIDgency to help you get settled. Then consider counseling to heal emotional wounds from the past and to provide you with skills for the future.

KEEPING YOUR SECRET AND PARENTING YOUR BABY

As mentioned before, most women who keep their pregnancies secret choose adoption. Some, however, make plans for parenting their babies themselves. Do you want to do this? Think carefully before you decide. Unless you are in a very difficult, unusual, or dangerous situation, it's much better to tell the truth. People will adjust in time.

However, if parenting your baby while keeping your pregnancy a secret is your only real choice, you must plan very carefully. You need an excuse for going away. Then you must fabricate an adoption story. You'll have to be strongly motivated to carry this off without telling complicated lies that might ensnare you. Below are some stories you could use.

- You could tell people that your parents have consented to adopt a relative's baby. Make up an excuse for going away. Send your newborn, known as the "relative's baby" to others, home. Then return home several months later.

    If you want to breastfeed, ask a PREGNANCY AIDgency to place your baby with a nearby family. You return home. Visit and breastfeed your baby daily until you bring the infant home several months later.

- Ask a close friend to parent your baby for a time. Tell people that this friend is helping out a friend or relative who can't parent right now. After a time, the baby's fabricated mother either dies or puts the baby up for adoption. Your friend doesn't wish to adopt the baby, but you have come to know and love the child. You decide to "adopt" the infant.

- You might tell people that you are making private adoption arrangements. Things are moving along quite quickly. However, you have to go away for a while on business or for some other fabricated reason.

    Find someone to parent your child temporarily. Leave your baby with this person and return home. In a few months, joyfully announce that your adoption has come through! You return to your baby's temporary home and bring the baby back with you, having "adopted" your child.

- You could say nothing about adoption. Instead, remark that a very ill relative or friend has been in touch with you. Get a friend or PREGNANCY AIDgency volunteer to play the role of this imaginary woman. Write her letters and telephone her.

    This woman eventually asks you to come and care for her, so you leave your family to do so. What you are really doing is going away to give birth. Finally, you agree to raise this woman's baby because she is too ill or emotionally unstable to do so. You might even say the woman died.

RECORD THE TRUTH

If you are planning to "adopt" your own baby, you need not sign any legal papers because the adoption is only a story. However, someone may question the adoption. Someday your child may want to find his or her "birth mother." Confidentially file the true story with your lawyer. Someday, when your present situation has passed, someone may need to know the facts.

> *At a dance, a married acquaintance offered Sarah, who had a physical disability, a ride home and raped her on the way. Single and pregnant, Sarah went to a maternity home but was so uncomfortable choosing adoption that her parents agreed to raise baby Ria as if she were Sarah's sister.*
>
> *Afraid that Ria would run away if she knew the truth, Ria's family did not tell her who her birth mother really was until she had come home from law school to care for the two elderly "parents," now terminally ill. When Sarah's mother told Ria that she was not Ria's mother, Ria gently responded, "I know. Sarah is. Someone told me years ago."*
>
> *After her "parents" died, Ria returned to law school. Today she has a successful law practice. Sarah lives with Ria. The two are very close.*

KEEPING THINGS QUIET

Pregnancies can be kept secret if they must be. Review your reasons for wanting to keep your pregnancy a secret. Are they strong enough to warrant the suggestions in this chapter? If so, enlist the help of someone you can trust plus your local PREGNANCY AIDgency. If you are strongly motivated, you can keep this pregnancy a secret from those who don't need to know, while still giving birth.

> *"In the midst of every hurricane lies a center of calm."*
>
> —*M.P.N.*

Relieving Panic and Stress

Does this pregnancy really worry you? You may be unable to think, eat, or sleep. You may feel as if you are losing your mind. Is this stress normal? Yes!

HORMONAL CHANGES PRODUCE STRESSFUL EMOTIONS

Pregnancy changes your body chemistry with hormones. Hormones are chemicals made by endocrine glands. They are secreted directly into your bloodstream. While keeping you pregnant, these pregnancy hormones also cause mood shifts regardless of whether your pregnancy involves crisis. This is why you may feel confident one minute and despairing the next. You're experiencing the normal emotional roller coaster of pregnancy. As your body adjusts to pregnancy, the hormonal upheaval will end and your moods will stabilize. Then you'll feel better!

If you're at the very beginning or very end of your childbearing years, your hormones will be even more disturbed. Even if you are not pregnant, your fluctuating level of hormones during adolescence and menopause can make you feel conspicuous, emotional, and irritable. This is how women who are entering puberty and menopause feel. Rebellion and depression are normal and will subside in time.

CRISIS CREATES UPHEAVAL

It takes a while to accept the fact that you really and truly are pregnant. When denial disappears, you'll feel emotions that range from worry to despair. How can this be happening? How can life go on normally when you are so tense and jumpy? Are people staring at you? How do you handle anger, guilt, fear, worry, helplessness, and frustration? Do you punch walls, run a marathon, cry? Will you ever smile again?

You may feel exhausted, nauseated, or tearful. You may experience cramps. Concentrating on anything seems impossible. You think only about yourself.

You're experiencing the normal symptoms of stress and adjustment. Experiencing strong emotions means that you are facing, not burying, your crisis. That's healthy.

SUICIDAL FEELINGS

You might get so depressed that you think of killing yourself. If you have these thoughts often, or if you are really considering suicide, call a suicide hotline, emergency helpline, or PREGNANCY AIDgency twenty-four-hour hotline. Call *now*! Chapter Seven has additional information on dealing with suicidal tendencies that you may have during your pregnancy.

THE EFFECT OF PAST TRAUMAS

Your past affects your self-image and your behavior. You may have unhealthy attitudes that are keeping you from handling this crisis well.

Physical, sexual, or emotional abuse or neglect can leave you feeling worthless. If no one seemed to care about you in the past, you may doubt that anyone will care now. Why should anyone care anyway? Why care yourself?

Perhaps in the past—or now—you did not "fit in" with your peers, and had few friends. Because of that, you may dislike yourself and feel incapable of dealing with others. You may be terrified of how others will react now that you are pregnant.

On the other hand, you may want to please your peer group. You may feel that popularity comes from "fitting in" and "going along with the crowd," and your crowd may think that giving birth is foolish.

Maybe you were hurt when someone said or did something to you or when someone you loved disappeared from your life. Perhaps you feel responsible, possibly unreasonably so, for being hurt. You may be afraid that this pregnancy will hurt others or you.

Perhaps you grew up in a home where a parent, grandparent, or guardian had addictions or other unhealthy life patterns. Did this person drink too much, abuse drugs, gamble, overeat, nurse depression, or have excessive or deviant sexual interests? Did this person break promises, overreact, or seem self-centered? This may have affected your self-esteem in a negative way. Or did this person give you everything you wanted and let you do as you pleased? This may have caused you to grow up thinking that life is supposed to be constantly easy.

We learn coping skills from our parents. If your grandparents had childish behaviors, your parents probably learned similar behaviors and parented you poorly. You learn from your parents. You may never have learned responsibility or maturity because no one in your family ever modeled those behaviors.

An indifferent, inconsistent, overly indulgent, overly restrictive, or abusive parent or guardian can make you feel helpless, incompetent, or rebellious. Because of your upbringing, it may be easy for others to manipulate you. You may try to run from a crisis. Perhaps you would rather do nothing than deal with a crisis.

THE EFFECT OF ADDICTIONS

If you're addicted to drugs, alcohol, gambling, spending, sex, food, or anything else, or if you engage in self-mutilation, you're running from your life or trying to bury emotional wounds. Why are you doing this? Peer pressure? An unhappy home life? School pressures? Stress? Is your addiction enjoyable?

Your maturity ends when your addiction begins. In order to plan for your baby, you need to think clearly and maturely. Stopping your addictive behavior definitely helps.

However, you can't break an addiction on your own. You need help. Take these three steps first: admit that you have an addiction, that you desperately want to stop the addiction permanently, and that you cannot stop it without help.

Understand your addiction. Appendix I lists some books that deal with addictions. Call a hospital or helpline for referral to counselors, psychologists, or self-help groups that deal with addictions. Appendix H lists some groups. If your area has no group that deals with your specific addiction, find a support group that focuses on a different addiction. Most "anonymous" groups follow the same twelve-step program. You'll find help, advice, and group support in staying "clean and serene" and in breaking your addiction. Then you will be able to plan a better life for yourself and your baby.

CONFIDE IN SOMEONE

Speak to someone who can help you work through your past and your problems while supporting your decision to bear your baby. How about your confidant? What about a counselor, member of the clergy, or self-help group? Consult books. Appendix I has some sources to help you. Discover in what areas you need healing and growth, and learn to deal with crisis.

Valerie came from a cold, uncommunicative, alcoholic, wealthy family. She had experienced the death of a sister, had experimented with drugs, and had several sexual relationships and three abortions. Despite a doctor's advice to abort, she had borne one child and was pregnant again. When this child was born severely ill, her mother-in-law, who disapproved of Valerie's racial background, committed suicide.

The product of a traumatic childhood, Valerie's husband had emotional problems, too. At Valerie's insistence, he stopped seeing other women, got a vasectomy, and went for counseling. Valerie began attending religious services, prayed daily, and sought spiritual counseling.

Today Valerie and her husband have a close relationship, although they are still working through some past traumas. Valerie is a family therapist specializing in Post Abortion Stress Syndrome and the medical aspects of abortion.

MANAGING STRESS

Regardless of whether you have experienced past traumas or have addictions, you must learn to manage stress or stress will manage you! You can manage stress in several ways, some of which are suggested here. Do whatever seems to work for you.

Physical Activity

Physical activity and exercise release stress. Because you're pregnant, you must be careful not to strain your abdominal muscles. Avoid pulling, stretching, heavy lifting, and other activities that put strain on your abdomen. Abdominal strain may harm you and your baby.

Always check with your doctor before engaging in sports or other physical activities, including those suggested here. If you have a health problem or have had a difficult previous pregnancy, your doctor may tailor an exercise program to fit your situation.

Ask your doctor about walking. It tones your body by strengthening your cardiovascular system and by exercising nearly all your muscles. You should jog only if you are a seasoned jogger, and only under a doctor's supervision. Walking and jogging get you outdoors, where the soothing psychological effects of natural light can help you feel better, too.

Indoors, you can walk in place, about fifty-five steps a minute. Do this for twenty minutes a day while watching TV, and you'll feel better.

All standard swimming strokes—crawl, breast stroke, side stroke—are usually fine during pregnancy. Check with your doctor to be sure. Swim a half mile or less daily in comfortably warm water.

Riding a regular bicycle is dangerous late in pregnancy, because your pregnant body changes your balance and you may fall. Bike stores sell equipment that can convert a regular bike into a stationary one. Or, you can buy or borrow a sturdy new or used stationary bike. Pedal for ten minutes, two or three times daily, at a comfortable rate of about seven miles per hour. You can buy a reading rack for a stationary bike and read while riding, or you can watch television while you ride.

Several books contain exercises for pregnant women, and a few are listed at the end of this book. Obtain these books from a library, doctor, or bookstore. Another good idea is to take prenatal exercise classes or prenatal aerobics. Look in your newspaper for details, or call your local hospital.

Relaxation Exercises

Ask your doctor about the following anti-stress exercise, suggested in many books on pregnancy fitness. Lie comfortably on your side with a pillow under your head. Keep your bottom leg relaxed and straight. Use two pillows to support your upper leg, comfortably bent at the knee. Late in pregnancy, you may use soft pillows to support your uterus or breasts. In this position, your body can be totally comfortable and relaxed.

Beginning with one foot, contract (tense or tighten up) that foot's muscles as *slowly* and tightly as possible while breathing in deeply and *slowly* through your nose. Then *slowly* relax your foot completely while breathing out *slowly* through your mouth. Think "contract" while contracting and "relax" while relaxing. Then *slowly* contract and relax your other foot.

Proceed *slowly* through each muscle in your body in the following order: each calf muscle (the muscle between your ankle and your knee), each thigh muscle (the muscle in your upper leg), your pelvic floor muscle (the muscle you use to stop urination), your buttocks, your abdomen, your chest, your shoulders, each hand, each arm, your neck, and your entire face. The more slowly you do these exercises, the more relaxed you will feel.

After finishing the exercises, take two *slow, deep* breaths through your nose and let them out *slowly* through your mouth.

Do relaxation exercises at least three times daily. You will soon be able to relax consciously. If you practice now, you will be able to do relaxation exercises during labor, and you will probably have a quicker, more comfortable delivery.

Housework

Your doctor will probably agree that nonstrenuous housework offers a safe, effective method for reducing tension, while completing disagreeable or boring tasks. Don't do anything that will strain your abdominal muscles or that might throw you off balance and cause a fall. Don't move or lift heavy items or climb on ladders and chairs! Avoid using disinfectants, furniture polishes, and other cleansers with strong fumes. It is usually safe to do light yard work, light housecleaning, and creative cooking.

Hobbies and Other Pursuits

Hobbies are excellent ways to relax. Unless you like to skydive or water-ski, most hobbies are safe to engage in during pregnancy. To be sure, ask your doctor.

Arts and crafts are fun. Don't worry about whether you're good at your craft. The goal is to relax and release tension, not to win a contest. Be sure to check with a doctor before using any paints or glues with strong fumes. Fumes can make you ill and may be harmful to your baby.

Techniques for Releasing Tension

Besides exercise and hobbies, there are some unusual tension-releasing methods that can be effective. The suggestions that follow may help.

- Scream—either out loud or in silence. But keep in mind that unborn babies four months old or older can hear your voice, so you may want to muffle your screams so as not to startle your child. Scream into a pillow, or turn on the bathroom shower full blast, and scream or sing at the top of your lungs.
- Punching pillows releases explosive anger and frustration and is much better than punching people or walls! It also helps if you have a tendency to harm yourself when you are upset. If your children catch you punching pillows, explain that you are upset, but not with them, and that this makes you feel better.
- Take a handful of newspaper and twist, tear, puncture, and shred it to bits. Cleaning up also reduces tension (whereas not cleaning up creates it!).
- Crying is a wonderful outlet for your emotions. A good cry may make you feel better.
- Do isometric exercises with your face, hands, and feet (do not do them with your abdomen or chest). Get comfortable. Contract your muscles as tightly as possible, in one area of your body at a time, then consciously relax them.

Quiet Relaxation Techniques

Relaxation is important for your health and that of your baby, and helps release tension. There are many things you can do to help yourself relax.

Don't overlook gentle touching. Ask a friend for a hug, a massage, or a back rub. Then return the favor. Have someone brush your hair. Touch and play with a pet. Cuddle a youngster or that special someone! Touching and being touched can help release stress from your body.

Take a warm shower. The flow of warm water and the murmur of the shower will put you at ease.

Get your sleep! This means seven or eight hours at night and a catnap or two during the day as well. Drink a glass of milk before going to bed. It acts as a natural tranquilizer. Or substitute cheese, low-calorie ice cream, or yogurt.

Watch Your Diet

Remember that whatever you put into your body affects both you and your baby. Some foods increase tension and nervousness, and have other undesirable effects.

Caffeine can make you "jumpy," absorb B vitamins, and increase your nausea. Avoid caffeine-containing foods, such as coffee, tea, chocolate, and many soft drinks, as well as chocolate- or coffee-flavored foods.

Pastries, candies, desserts, soft drinks, and many breakfast cereals contain excess sugar. Sugar's quick pick-up takes a quick downturn to exhaustion and depression.

Many processed foods, mixes, candies, pastries, and dry cereals contain artificial colors, flavors, and preservatives. If you are sensitive to these additives, you'll feel jumpy, frustrated, sleepless, angry, or depressed for hours or even days after eating them.

One in ten people has a food sensitivity but does not know it. If you have a food allergy, you may feel ill, tense, or grouchy after eating the offensive food. Appendix I lists some books that can help you discover food allergies and tell you how to handle them.

Avoid alcoholic beverages, smoking, overeating, and taking drugs. These are bad for you and your baby, can cause addictions, and can mask your problems without really helping you to solve them. Find better ways to relax.

BURNOUT

Heavy involvement in your career or in home, school, social, or civic activities, coupled with pregnancy worries, may make you feel as if you are losing or out of control. You may be burning yourself out by trying to do too much.

With your confidant, evaluate your lifestyle and what you should do. You may need to make some changes.

If you feel as if you are doing too much, reduce your activities. Re-examine your hectic schedule and keep only those activities that give you the most satisfaction. Learn to say "no" to requests for your time. Each day, consciously take some time to relax. Each week, do something that you really enjoy. Make lists of jobs you would like done, do what's important, and let the rest go. Admit that you cannot do *everything* well at the same time.

BE CALM

You can help yourself calm down. As your pregnant body's rapid hormonal shifts slow down and attain an equilibrium, you will begin to feel better. As you start to manage your life, you'll feel calmer, too. Each day, do something to reduce your tension. As you feel calmer, you'll be able to deal more rationally with your future, think more clearly, and make workable plans. Meeting these objectives is cause for rejoicing!

> *Doubt sees the obstacles—*
> *Faith sees the way!*
> *Doubt sees the darkest night—*
> *Faith sees the day!*
> *Doubt dreads to take a step—*
> *Faith soars on high.*
> *Doubt questions, "Who Believes?"—*
> *Faith answers, "I."*
>
> *—Author unknown*

Developing a Positive Attitude

Remember the familiar children's story *The Little Engine That Could?* The little engine faced the almost impossible task of pulling a much larger disabled train over a high mountain. The little engine chugged up the mountain, chanting, "I think I can. I think I can." And she succeeded because she worked hard and thought positively.

When you talk to yourself (and we all do that—quietly or out loud), what do you say? Do you make plans with confidence or are you a negative thinker? Do you think, "I can *never* solve this problem" or "I *can't* do it" or "This will *never* work out"? If so, negative thinking paralyzes you!

You must learn to think positively. "I *can* solve this problem." "I *can* do it." "This *will* work out." "I think I can" will help you get the job done. Positive thinking really does work. Try it. You'll be surprised at how good you'll start to feel about yourself.

BECOME A POSITIVE THINKER

You will have to keep reminding yourself to be a positive thinker. Below are some suggestions by Robert Handley, an expert in positive thinking.

- Stick colorful children's stickers in various locations such as on your refrigerator, typewriter, phone, and notebook. Whenever you see a sticker, examine whether you feel relaxed and what you are thinking. Are you tense? Are you engaging in negative self-talk?
- If you're tense, relax following a technique mentioned previously in this chapter. Change any negative thoughts into positive ones. If you're thinking, "I can't do this," think instead, "I can do this." If you're nervous, tell yourself, "I can feel calm." If you feel that your situation is hopeless, think, "This will work out."
- Visualize yourself working successfully through your problems. Visualize how you would act, what you would say, who you would see, where you would be, and what you would have to do to make this vision a reality. Let this book guide you.
- Act like the person you want to be. Act peaceful and confident, even if you're nervous, and you will influence your subconscious mind. You will actually start to become a more confident, calm woman.
- Avoid people who tell you that you can't handle your life and who feed you other negative thoughts. They will undermine your confidence.
- Find inspirational books in a library, bookstore, church, or synagogue, or borrow some. If you read ten or fifteen minutes a day, your outlook will brighten.
- Whenever you do something to build your confidence, congratulate yourself. Say, "Great job! You did it!" or a similar praiseworthy comment.

TREAT YOURSELF WELL

Gain perspective by "getting away from it all." When you return from your "vacation," you will feel more relaxed and better able to cope. If you can't afford to pay for a vacation, consider a brief visit to a relative or friend who lives in another area.

If you are financially able to do so, take an actual vacation in an enjoyable location with a minimum of stress. Stay as long as possible. Do what feels comfortable. Check with a doctor to see what kinds of physical activity are advisable.

Go on a retreat. Religious groups allow individuals who pay a minimal fee to visit retreat houses for periods of time. Meals and a bedroom are provided. Counselors are available if you want to talk. Even if you aren't "religious," you can still "make a retreat." Retreats can be made in groups or alone. No one will try to convert you! It will help you immensely just to get away. If you like, you can seek out individuals who can encourage you. If you don't want company, you will be left alone. Local churches and synagogues may be able to direct you to a nearby retreat center.

For a few hours, enjoy a quiet spot of natural beauty and gain perspective. Watch the sunset or sunrise or lie beneath the stars. Your problems will seem smaller.

Do you have pretty house plants, an aquarium, or a flower garden? Get into a comfortable position and simply meditate on the loveliness of nature. If you don't own any living thing, purchase a plant or a pretty dried flower arrangement to use as a meditative focal point. When close to nature, we see our problems in a more realistic way.

Try to do something nice for yourself every day. Even if you only read a short poem, play a relaxing record, or have a cool glass of juice, give yourself a little treat and learn to relax for a moment or two. Once a week, treat yourself to something special. You'll soon begin to feel better.

DO FOR OTHERS

When you feel washed out, depressed, and confused, you may wonder how you can give anything to others. But, as long as you don't overcommit yourself, doing something for someone else often helps to put your own problems in perspective. It lets you see that others are in need, too.

Find a religious or community group that helps others. Volunteer at a nursing home, school, thrift shop, soup kitchen, or hospital. Visit a lonely person. Play with a child. Shop for a shut-in. Pray for someone. Do someone an unexpected favor. It's easy to find someone in need. Brightening another's day will brighten yours, too.

Of course, thinking about what you are doing for your baby can help you feel good, too. Your child will have a good life because of your plans.

KEEP YOUR SENSE OF HUMOR

A famous person once said, "To laugh is to jog internally." Laughing really helps, both your body and your attitude.

Now it may seem cruel or ridiculous for someone to tell you to keep your sense of humor when you are in a pregnancy crisis. Your whole future seems to be spinning away! What's funny about that?

In the midst of every crisis should be something bright and light. If you cannot find anything at all, speak to a counselor. You may need to live elsewhere, in a more peaceful, comfortable, and joyful environment. Only then can you deal with the seriousness of your crisis.

What can you laugh about? You might laugh at your mistakes, about how you've changed, and about how you've taken life so seriously. Read a joke book, a funny story, or the daily comics. Watch a genuinely humorous movie, video, or television show. See a comedy in the theater. Go to a playground or zoo and watch the children. If you like to play on the playground equipment or go to an amusement park, ask your doctor if you can. Remember, you're pregnant, so avoid jolting, jerking, and wild rides.

Laughter is medicine for the soul. Look for the odd, funny, and unexpected. Make yourself smile again.

Lynn and Fred planned on having four children. During her fifth pregnancy, Lynn joked about her "surprise package," who was really a surprise when he was born on the way to the hospital. When Lynn got pregnant with number six, she said, "What's one more?" and was glad that her youngest would have a playmate.

For an hour a day, Lynn has the older children babysit the younger ones, giving Lynn time to herself. She attends a weekly prayer meeting. Fred gets up an hour early and has that time to read or walk outdoors. Fred and Lynn often go out on a "date," without the kids along.

Lynn and Fred have stopped trying to be perfect. They saved time by switching to convenience foods and work-saving gardening methods. The older children "clean" their rooms (Lynn keeps their bedroom doors closed!), and Lynn cleans less frequently.

Lynn and Fred are able to handle and enjoy their busy, large family because they divide up work, laugh about their frustrations, and take time for themselves.

YOU'RE GONNA MAKE IT!

Success doesn't come just because we think it will. Yet success hardly ever comes if we think it won't! Usually only those who think they will succeed do.

Remember Dumbo the elephant? He could fly—he certainly had huge enough ears. Yet he didn't believe in himself. He could fly only when his mouse friend gave him a "magic" feather.

Dumbo became the star of the circus. Then, one day, while Dumbo was soaring, the feather slipped out of his trunk. Realizing that the feather was gone, Dumbo panicked and began to fall. His mouse friend shouted, "You can fly! It wasn't a magic feather. You can fly. Try!"

Faced with death from crashing into the ground below, Dumbo tried. He really could fly! The feather was just a mental crutch.

Maybe you're used to seeing yourself as a "dumbo." You're not used to believing in yourself. Now is the time to begin! Every "dumbo" has gifts and talents.

Use yours now. When you think positively, you'll be surprised at what you can decide and do.

"One good plan is worth ten million regrets."

—*M.P.N.*

Writing Your Way Through Your Crisis

If you hate to write, the idea of a journal might give you a headache! But a journal is more than a diary or essay. A journal is a tool for defining your problems and organizing and meeting your needs. A well-kept journal will reduce your tension, not increase it. And a journal is only for you. No one else has to read it, so you can write whatever you want.

Lots of women get through their pregnancy crisis without a journal. However, some of these women would have managed better had they kept a journal.

On the other hand, lots of women do keep journals. Ruth Heil kept one during each of her five pregnancies. Then she turned her journals into a book, *My Child Within*.

Will keeping a journal help you? Try it and decide.

How long should you keep a journal? As long as it's helpful. Some days you may write much in your journal; other days, nothing. How much you use your journal depends on you and your situation.

HOW TO KEEP A JOURNAL

A journal is simply a notebook. Begin filling the blank pages by writing down the emotions or symptoms (such as frustration, anger, guilt, loneliness, helplessness, fear, depression, or weakness) you feel, one emotion or symptom to one page, and the day's date.

When you finish that, go back and look at what you've written. Under each emotion or symptom write the problem that causes it. This will help you understand what is bothering you. You may not realize what is on your mind.

Be thorough. Write down *everything* that is bothering you. At least you'll *know* why you are upset, and writing may inspire some solutions.

Be patient. For a few days, don't attempt to solve your problems or make snap decisions. Just record your emotions or symptoms and your problems whenever you think of them. Then you can start to solve them.

After writing down your problems for a few days, reread your journal. As you do, encourage yourself with positive self-talk. Write it down!

Here is a sample journal page that shows how recording your emotions can lead to defining your problems.

June 5—I'm scared.

I think I'm pregnant. If I am, I might lose my job. I'll embarrass Mom and Dad. What about the gossip? I hate to be talked about. And what will Daddy do?

June 7—Today I'll encourage myself. I can handle pregnancy. I'm twenty years old. It's not as if I don't know about life. If I embarrass people, then I embarrass them. I can make it. I can stand gossip. I can handle Daddy. If I don't like what he tries to do, I can leave. Things are going to be all right.

Define Your Needs

Think about what you've written. Can you discover what you need to solve your problems? Your confidant may be able to help.

For example, if you are worried about your family's reaction to this pregnancy, you will need to formulate a plan to tell them. You may need to live someplace else. You may even decide to conceal your pregnancy.

Write each need on a separate page of the journal, starting each page with the words "I would like" or "I could use." Also record the date.

Each woman's needs differ. Take several days to define your needs, then reread them. Do they accurately reflect your concerns?

Put Your Needs in Order

After you've used your journal to define your needs, you can refer to what you've written and divide your needs into several categories.

What needs should be met as soon as possible? One vital, immediate need is medical care, and you may also need other professional advice. It might be helpful for you to obtain emotional support, and you may wish to see a PREGNANCY AIDgency as well. You will probably want to find a confidant.

What needs have to be met soon, but not immediately? Perhaps you don't want anyone to know about your pregnancy. In that case, it might be good for you to relocate elsewhere, but you don't have to move this weekend. You have time to plan.

What decisions have to be made, but can be put off until the very end of pregnancy or even after birth? You have ample time before making a final decision regarding adoption or a decision about resuming your career once the baby is born.

Which things would you like to do, but could live without if you had to? Perhaps you want to attend your school prom, but it is scheduled right around your due date—you can go if you're not in labor or the delivery room! Or you may have a passion to learn skydiving that is best put off until after your baby is born!

As you read through this book, you'll find it easier to separate immediate needs from future ones. In a pregnancy crisis, it's definitely better to put off until tomorrow what doesn't have to be done today. This doesn't mean that you shouldn't plan ahead, but it does mean you should take one day at a time.

If necessary, conceal your pregnancy so that you can postpone dealing with some situations until you are ready. Work out how to meet future needs later on. Right now, concentrate on the needs that must be met now.

If you have problems ordering your needs according to their urgency, ask for help from a trusted friend, counselor, PREGNANCY AIDgency volunteer, or member of the clergy.

Record Vital Information

You will need to remember the phone numbers, addresses, locations, fees, and business hours of agencies, doctors, childbirth classes, shelters, and counselors, and any appointments you have with them. If you have specific prescriptions or vitamins to take, record that information. You may need to request maternity leave or to reschedule plans.

Record all specific information in your journal under the need you are meeting. That way, vital information will be at your fingertips. Everything you need to know will be in your journal. Just make sure you keep it in a safe place and don't lose it!

Meet Your Needs

The remainder of this book discusses how to meet the specific needs of your pregnancy crisis. Once you have used your journal to define just what you need, you can refer to the sections of this book that discuss your specific needs. As you look through this book, you may think of other needs as well. Continue to record your needs as soon as you understand them, and to date your journal entries. Think positively about your ability to obtain what you need. Check the dates recorded in your journal to see how far you've already come. Encourage yourself!

Here is a sample journal page that shows how one woman defined a problem, classified it as an immediate need, and went about meeting that need.

Immediate Problem to Solve

June 8—I want to find out for sure if I am pregnant.

Looked in phone book. Birthright—777-7777. Appointment for June 10. 12:00 p.m. (my lunch hour).

June 10—Yep. Pregnancy test is positive. My volunteer counselor, Flo, is really nice. I can trust and confide in her as a friend. She told me I could go live in a shelter home and tell Mom I was taking a secretarial course. A secretary can teach me when I'm there. Then I can make an adoption plan for my baby, without Mom knowing, if I want to. I have to think about that.

Flo also gave me the name of a doctor—Dr. Hayes. Appointment with him, 34 Beech Street, June 17, 4:45 p.m. 681-2349. Will tell Mom I went to the mall to get pantyhose.

June 17—Dr. Hayes is nice. Prenatal vitamin prescription at Grimes Pharmacy, 465 Main Street. Open 24 hours. Will hide vitamins in my bureau drawer so Mom doesn't find them. Next appointment with Dr. Hayes—July 21, 4:45 p.m. Call first to make sure he's not delivering a baby. I can't believe this is working out at last.

USE YOUR PLAN

You're creating a plan for your pregnancy crisis! This plan is going to work, and you are capable of seeing that it does. By wisely using your journal, you can define your needs. This book will help you meet them.

One knot today. One knot tomorrow. Some knots will be easy to untangle, others will be more difficult. Some knots will untangle after a single phone call, and others will take months to straighten out. But you can untangle every knot you face in the jumble that seemed so hopeless a short while ago.

Right now you may not know exactly what you are creating. However, as you untangle your crisis, you can be sure that you are knitting its threads into something new and beautiful.

> *"You cannot escape necessities;*
> *but you can conquer them."*
>
> —*Seneca*

Obtaining the Essentials

All pregnant women have similar, basic needs: food, clothing, shelter, and medical care. This section will help you define and meet some of these needs.

FEEL WELL

Many minor physical complaints often accompany pregnancy. Deal with them and you will feel better.

- If you tire easily, get to bed early and catnap during the day.
- If you get skin rashes, ask your doctor or pharmacist for a lotion or cream that is safe to use during pregnancy.
- Sleep on your side or back and buy a bra in a larger size to ease the pain of swollen, sore breasts.
- To control heartburn and belching, eliminate spicy foods, eat slowly, and don't overeat.
- If you get a leg cramp, immediately get up and walk until the cramp disappears.
- Wear support stockings to help varicose veins.
- If you have an irritating or itchy vaginal discharge, ask your doctor for medication and wear a thin menstrual pad or an extra pair of cotton panties.
- If you urinate frequently, continue to drink water and fruit juices for good bowel regulation—but stay close to a toilet!
- If you have constipation or diarrhea, ask your doctor for a diet to control these conditions.
- If you have morning sickness, try munching on saltine crackers, dry toast, or dry cereal before you even get out of bed. Then, get up slowly. Eat small, frequent meals, rest a bit after eating, and keep a small amount of food in your stomach. Don't skip meals. Avoid spicy and greasy foods and foods you used to love that now make you ill. Suck lollipops or hard candies. Or make ice pops from fruit juice frozen in paper cups, and stick in a spoon for a handle.
- Talk to your doctor about prenatal vitamins and a vitamin B supplement or injection, both of which might control nausea. Your doctor can manage severe

nausea medically. A mild tranquilizer prescribed by a doctor will make you feel better if stress is making you ill.

EAT WELL

Proper diet is essential for your health and the health of your baby. The following guidelines will help you plan and maintain good eating habits.

- Follow a sensible diet. Choose natural, unprocessed foods. Cut down on salty, sugary, and fatty foods. Don't overdo on starches and carbohydrates.
- For a well-balanced diet that can meet the demands of pregnancy, consult your doctor. Your diet should include dairy products, meats, fish, fruits, vegetables, breads, and cereals. You can treat yourself now and then to a frankfurter, cupcake, or soft drink. However, a steady diet of high-calorie, low-nutrition foods will put on unnecessary weight and provide few nutrients.
- If you cannot afford to buy nutritious food, consult government agencies for assistance. Government aid may also help you obtain prenatal vitamins, another necessity for good health during pregnancy.
- Teens often have premature, unhealthy babies because teenaged moms often eat very poor diets. Eat wisely and your baby will probably be fine.
- If you've been dieting, the idea of gaining weight during pregnancy may make you feel faint! A doctor will help you develop a good diet so that the weight you gain will come off easily and quickly after you give birth.
- If you're anorexic or bulimic, see a doctor and a psychologist at once. Anorexia and bulimia are dangerous conditions and need professional management.
- If you're trying to keep your pregnancy a secret, don't starve yourself to stay thin. Instead, eat well, wear concealing clothing, and tell everyone that you're on a health food kick.
- Don't drink alcoholic beverages, smoke, or take drugs—these habits are bad for both you and your baby.

Saving Money on Food

Natural foods stores and groceries carry many affordable, nutritious foods. Buy store-brand and generic items instead of name brands. Plan menus around foods on sale. Use coupons only if you need the food item and only if the price, minus coupon savings, is cheaper than any other brand of the same food.

Instead of buying relatively expensive processed foods, mixes, or heat-and-serve dishes, use a good cookbook to make simple, nutritious meals from scratch. If you don't cook, ask a friend or neighbor to teach you how.

Buy basic cooking equipment cheaply at garage sales, thrift shops, and store sales. Make sure it's not damaged and is made of safe materials. A doctor or consumer protection group may be able to advise you. Grow your own vegetables or buy some from a home vegetable gardener. Stop buying nonessentials such as cigarettes, alcohol, sweets, snack foods, soft drinks, coffee, gum, and pastries.

Addictions to drugs, alcohol, and even cigarettes are dangerous and costly. Use clinics and self-help groups to help you overcome any addictions.

Feeding the Baby

Feeding your baby doesn't need to be expensive. The following suggestions will help you with this area.

- Breastfeeding your baby is cheaper than buying formula. Breastfeeding groups or nurses can tell you how to store breast milk for your baby if you are working outside the home.
- If you must use formula, government assistance may pay for it. If you are not eligible, a PREGNANCY AIDgency may be able to provide free formula.
- Make your own baby food using a special, inexpensive baby food grinder or a blender. Baby care books, nurses, and mothers' groups can tell you how to do this so your baby will be healthy.
- Ask your doctor or pharmacist to recommend a good, inexpensive children's vitamin. Vitamins keep your child healthier and cut down on visits to the doctor.

HOUSING OPTIONS

Shelter means a supportive, relaxed environment where you can think positively about yourself, your baby, and your future. If you're not in such a home, you may want to relocate. Perhaps you can live with a friend or relative.

Some of the agencies listed in the back of this book can refer you to maternity homes and group shelters. Each maternity home provides shelter for several pregnant women, sometimes for a fee. If you can't pay, many homes will drop the fee.

Free group shelter facilities house homeless women and their children, usually for a short time only. A social service agency can refer you to women's shelters.

A PREGNANCY AIDgency can house you with a family in a "shelter home." You can choose the location of this home, either in your community or elsewhere. You and the family must be able to get along. The family will treat you as a family member and expect you to help around the house a bit. You may be able to stay with some families for a few weeks after you give birth.

Housing for Minors

Each society has designated a certain age, usually in the upper teens, at which it considers a young person to be an adult. Call a government official, police officer, or school guidance counselor to find out the legal adult age. If you are older than this legal age, you can live anywhere you like. If you are under this age, you are considered a minor and different laws apply. A PREGNANCY AIDgency and lawyer can advise you.

Are you a minor living on your own? You may be considered an emancipated minor. You may be able to move elsewhere without parental consent.

Are you an abused minor? You may be eligible for a court-appointed guardian. Then you can possibly live away from home without your parent's consent.

Are you a minor living with your parent or legal guardian? Your parent or guardian will probably have to consent to your moving elsewhere during your pregnancy.

Permanent Housing

If you're not planning to return home to live, you'll need to find permanent housing. Perhaps you can afford to share an apartment with a friend or relative. Look in the rental columns of a newspaper or place an ad yourself. Interview all potential apartment mates—you need someone who will respect and encourage you.

Read the help-wanted ads. Someone may need live-in help. If they hire you, you will have a job, income, and home.

Government agencies can often refer you to low-income housing in your area. Or, you can move to an area where housing costs are low.

A PREGNANCY AIDgency or women's resource network may help you find housing and inexpensive furniture.

FURNITURE, CLOTHING, AND OTHER MATERIALS

If you can afford to buy everything you need brand-new, great! If not, save money by shopping at thrift shops, secondhand stores, and garage sales. Watch the newspaper's classified ads for used baby furniture, baby clothing, and maternity clothes. Go to an auction, listen to a radio "flea market" where callers advertise used items for sale, or shop in factory outlets. Borrow what you need from a friend or persuade someone to host a baby shower. Some PREGNANCY AIDgencies might give you free baby furniture, baby clothing, and maternity clothes. Check with a consumer protection group to see if all secondhand items meet government safety standards.

Be creative. A baby can get by without a lot of gadgets. However, you will need a car seat to keep your baby safe while you are driving. At home, be sure that your baby sleeps in a sturdy, safe place, such as a crib that meets current safety standards. If you're furnishing an apartment, consider doing it in "Early American Garage Sale"!

When three women living in different areas became pregnant, they could no longer live with their parents. Each of these women—Aster, Jessica, and Roxanna—sought housing through various agencies. After moving from tenement to hotel, Aster lived in a church-affiliated home for single mothers. Through a government agency, Jessica found a maternity home that helped her locate an apartment after her baby was born. A PREGNANCY AIDgency moved Roxanna, whose parents disapproved of her biracial love affair, into a low-rent apartment that was furnished with donated furniture. Various agencies provided these women with medical care, vocational training, government assistance, food aid, baby items, and training for parenthood.

SOURCES OF MONEY

If you *need* money, government assistance may help with medical expenses, food, and rent. You may be able to receive food stamps, heating assistance, aid to families with dependent children, free school lunches, and admittance to soup kitchens. This might be true even if you are not receiving government assistance. If you are receiving assistance, you may be due for an increase because of your pregnancy. If you are relocating, you should be able to receive assistance in your new area. A social service agency can advise you.

If you meet judgmental, rude, or harsh government workers, as Shelley did (Chapter Three), remember that you have a right to have your baby and receive assistance. It is illegal to cut back your welfare payment if you choose to give birth or don't consent to sterilization or abortion. A social service agency can help you deal with threats.

Private Sources of Financial Help

You may be in financial need yet ineligible for government funds because you are not a citizen or because of other factors. Perhaps government funds have been cut or are simply not enough. Call churches, PREGNANCY AIDgencies, charity groups, and possibly even your local newspaper's consumer rights reporter or features editor. A reporter might do an article on your desperate situation. See if a social service representative will write a letter to the editor about your situation.

A group may hold a fund raiser in your behalf. Someone may make an outright money gift. Churches may have "benevolent funds" that can give you money. Perhaps you can work part-time, even from your home, providing child care, filling mail orders, typing, or doing phone work (refer to the information on careers in Chapter Three). Cut back on nonessential expenses. If your financial situation is very bleak, you may choose to consider an adoption plan for your baby.

> *Both Alexandra and Lisa had huge bills to pay when they became pregnant.*
>
> *Alexandra was taking her two-month-old, breast-fed son with her while she worked two babysitting/housekeeping jobs to supplement her husband's meager paycheck. Lisa's husband was unemployed.*
>
> *Alexandra's doctor said breastfeeding while pregnant could have harmed her baby. This is highly unlikely. Lisa had health problems so serious that doctors thought she'd never get pregnant. When she did become pregnant, they predicted that she and her baby would have severe health problems. Both Alexandra and Lisa prayed that they would somehow find help.*
>
> *After using up a savings account to buy formula, Alexandra received government assistance. Two months later, her husband got a better job and Alexandra was able to quit hers.*
>
> *In despair, Lisa scheduled an abortion but met, outside the clinic, a pro-life sidewalk counselor who offered her free baby items and financial aid. Lisa accepted the help. Her husband got another job.*
>
> *Both women had smooth pregnancies and healthy babies whom they deeply love.*

If you are not a citizen and you wish to parent your baby, your baby will be a citizen and should be eligible for government assistance even if you are not.

How Will You Pay for the Doctor?

Who is going to pay the doctor, midwife, or hospital? If you're not eligible for government aid, a PREGNANCY AIDgency may be able to find a doctor and/or hospital to care for you free of charge or at very minimal cost. You will be able to pay back any bills over a long period of time. After a normal birth, you can save money by going home within twenty-four hours or even earlier, if you have someone at home to help you.

Home birth is less expensive than hospital birth and generally not risky if your pregnancy is normal. However, unforeseen and possibly dangerous problems can arise in any birth. Talk over the pros and cons of home birth with your doctor. Your doctor can also refer you to a midwife who conducts home births.

If you make an adoption plan, the adoption agency or adopting couple should pay your medical expenses.

LONG-RANGE FINANCIAL PLANNING

Social service agencies can refer you to a financial planner who may give you free budgeting advice. Books on financial planning can also help. You may have to learn to budget well if you're going to parent.

Earning a high school diploma, if you're without one, will get you a better job and higher pay.

Try to choose recreational activities that are not costly. Be creative. Visit parks and other free recreational places. Pack your own lunch instead of buying it in restaurants. Invite friends over for a bring-something-to-eat-with-you party. Give inexpensive gifts. Have fun by being with those you love without spending much money.

Unmarried and pregnant, seventeen-year-old Rheta lived in a cramped attic and worked as a maid. After her daughter's birth, she worked nights and studied for her high school equivalency diploma days while a neighbor babysat. Rheta continued working low-paying jobs and receiving welfare while she bore two sons. She moved into a low-income housing project and eventually obtained an associate's degree from a nearby college.

Rheta always took time to do simple, fun things with her children. She became involved with their school and sports events. Her two oldest children attended college, and her youngest is doing well in high school.

BEGINNING TO UNTANGLE YOUR CRISIS

Helping yourself means meeting certain basic needs. Start a good, healthy diet and obtain prenatal vitamins as soon as possible. You may be able to delay answering shelter and clothing concerns until later. If finances are a problem, much help is available from government and private agencies as well as PREGNANCY AIDgencies. If you want additional information on any topic, Appendix I lists many excellent sources to consult. Meeting basic needs is a good place to begin untangling your crisis.

Chapter Three

DEALING WITH OTHERS

"The M.D. after a doctor's name doesn't mean 'mostly divine.'"

—*M.P.N.*

Dealing Wisely With Professionals

Most professionals are caring, honest people who will treat you as a person with intelligence, rights, and feelings. Once they know you have a plan for your crisis, most will support your decision to give birth.

WHY DO PROFESSIONALS SUGGEST ABORTION?

Because some women have sued doctors for not mentioning abortion, most doctors will ask if you plan to have your baby. Say, "Of course I do." A caregiver who respects you will not question you further.

However, some caregivers imply that your only sensible option is abortion. Others may manipulate you toward, "lobby" for, or even insist on abortion. Why?

Some professionals think that any woman in pregnancy crisis should abort. Others think that women with large families or low incomes should not have children because they might be unable to care for them properly or they might be unable to pay their medical bills. Some are afraid of malpractice suits if the mother or baby has health problems. Others believe that babies with special needs, terminal illnesses, or fatal abnormalities should not be born. Still others simply don't want to bother with difficult pregnancies.

A nurse in a large metropolitan hospital, Yvette cared for a downcast, pregnant foreign woman who was extremely dehydrated due to severe pregnancy-related nausea. Although the woman's chart indicated that she was scheduled for an abortion, the woman told Yvette that she very much wanted her baby, but her doctor told her that she needed an abortion because she was so sick.

Yvette went to see the doctor. "You know she doesn't need an abortion," Yvette told him. "We manage nausea all the time. She'll be fine."

The doctor replied casually, "Oh, you don't know the women from this country. They think that the sicker they are, the healthier their babies will be. This woman will be sick the whole pregnancy. She'll always be in here."

The doctor's casual attitude stunned Yvette. She told the woman that she did not need an abortion. Did she still want to have her baby? The woman began to cry tears of gratitude. After treatment for nausea, she left the hospital still pregnant.

CHOOSING SUPPORTIVE PROFESSIONALS

Always remember—the choice to give birth to your baby is *yours*. Professionals cannot *force* you to have an abortion. However, they may try very hard to make you think it's the only sensible choice. It's not. Unless you will die if you give birth, you can probably have your baby without ruining your lifestyle, reputation, or future.

Friends, relatives, PREGNANCY AIDgencies, hospitals, nurses, or churches may be able to suggest competent professionals to call. A professional should, above all, have respect for your baby, your ability to manage during a crisis, and you.

Respect for Your Baby

Every professional should recognize that your unborn baby is an amazing human being (refer to Appendix A). A good doctor may let you hear your baby's heartbeat, acknowledge that babies can learn and respond before birth, and suggest that you talk to your child. A doctor should treat your child's special needs or terminal illness with the latest medical advances.

If you're like Beth, you'll be wary of doctors who are very casual about your baby's life. Of the four doctors she consulted about the effects surgery had had on her unborn baby before she realized that she was pregnant, three said that her baby was probably unharmed. The fourth commented, "If you're worried, just get an abortion." Beth chose one of the first three doctors she consulted. She delivered a healthy baby.

Respect for Your Ability to Manage a Crisis

Professionals should respect your plans to face your crisis. However, keep any information about your crisis to yourself, unless a professional needs to know it in order to treat you. Doctors, lawyers, and psychologists are not pregnancy counselors.

Suppose you mention the crisis or the professional knows about it. A professional should acknowledge that you have the intelligence and determination to make a well-devised plan and give birth. A professional who does not respect your abilities will try to tell you what to do. Jennifer's dentist was such a person.

When Jennifer became pregnant, her doctor stopped the medication she'd been taking for neuralgia, saying her baby would be fine. However, her dentist told her to abort the baby, "who must certainly be damaged." Jennifer bore a healthy child.

Respect for You

Professionals should respect you. Some professionals think that you should accept their suggestions without question. Be wary if your questions are answered with a pat on the hand and the words, "There, there, just trust us." You have a right to know *why* the plans they suggest are best for you and your baby and why they have rejected other alternatives. If you appear outwardly as someone whom others can manipulate, you will open yourself to the possibility of being manipulated.

> *Unexpectedly pregnant at forty-two, Faith and her husband consulted two doctors and dismissed the one who implied that Faith might as well abort. The doctor they chose encouraged the couple, laughing with them about "getting pregnant from the well water" and "being the oldest parents involved in Little League." Although depressed at first, Faith and her husband now immensely enjoy their son.*

HOW TO TALK TO PROFESSIONALS

In speaking to professionals, be assertive and firm but polite. Be positive about your decision to have your baby. If necessary, share the plans you're making for your baby's future and the information in this book.

If you are asked personal details that have no bearing on the professional's area of expertise, say, "That information is personal." If a caregiver says something disturbing or acts in a rude, discourteous, or patronizing manner, say, "What you've just said disturbs me," or "That tone of voice makes me uncomfortable," or "You seem to be dodging my questions, but I believe I have a right to know that information."

Professionals often ask questions simply to make "small talk" or to "put you at ease." Other pushy professionals have a "Dear Abby" complex and like to give advice! Of course, you needn't take it!

Appendix E contains questions you might ask professionals or yourself. Answers to these questions will help you identify just what you like, dislike, or hope to change about those who are working with you.

If someone else in your family needs medical, legal, or psychological help, you may use some of the guidelines in this chapter to find professionals to help.

> *Velma was glad when she found out she was pregnant, but her husband Emil worried about stretching family finances and became suicidal. A PREGNANCY AIDgency recommended a good psychiatrist who prescribed rest, medication, and counseling for Emil. Now Emil feels much better, worries less, and adores his son.*

YOUR "BILL OF RIGHTS"

The International Childbirth Education Association (ICEA) has prepared two excellent documents, the "Pregnant Patient's Bill of Rights" and "Pregnant Patient's Responsibilities." Many doctors and hospitals' obstetric units have copies. So do many childbirth books. You can also obtain a copy by writing to ICEA, P.O. Box 20048, Minneapolis, Minnesota 55420-0048, or by calling 612/854-8660. Your doctor and hospital should be familiar with and agree with these documents.

The "Pregnant Patient's Bill of Rights" explains that you have a right to full information about all treatments, procedures, and medications that your doctor suggests. You also have a right to refuse medications or procedures or to request alternate ones. The "Pregnant Patient's Responsibilities" points out that you are responsible for courteously communicating your preferences to your health care team and for listening to their reasons for suggested treatments. You are then responsible for following the treatments that you and your doctor have agreed upon. In determining a health care program, tell your doctor if you are already taking vitamins or medications or if you exercise, because these things may affect your treatment.

Discuss anything that is bothering you with your doctor. Between doctor's visits, write down your concerns and take your questions with you. Be sure they're answered.

CHANGING AND EDUCATING PROFESSIONALS

If you don't like the caregiver you have, choose another. If you must use a certain professional, or if you like many things but not everything about the individual, you can try to educate the person. Many women have brought professionals to their way of thinking. Use this book to help.

If you must deal with a negative thinker, say firmly, "I appreciate your concern, but I am definitely planning to have my baby and I've got the plans to do so under way. Please respect my judgment and the way I am handling my situation." Then refer to this book and to a trained pregnancy counselor for help. Rely on a positive-thinking confidant to encourage you.

Bernice received a German measles vaccination two weeks before getting pregnant. Three doctors told her to get an abortion; a fourth gave her a zero-percent chance of having a healthy baby. Bernice and her husband comforted each other and prayed that they would accept their baby, who was born perfectly healthy. They ignore those professionals, acquaintances, and family members who still say that Bernice should have had an abortion.

MAKING SURE YOUR BABY WILL BE BORN

What treatment would you want if you ever became mentally incompetent? Should your baby be saved even if you might die? What if your baby has special needs or a terminal illness?

In a recent two-year period, three of the United States' largest trauma centers treated a total of twenty pregnant women in comas. Other centers reported treating additional coma cases. Usually, the coma ended and the woman went home and had her baby. But that's not always what happens.

Both about three months pregnant, Diane and Goldie sustained severe brain damage in two different auto accidents. Both were in comas.

Diane's husband and mother had a doctor perform an abortion on Diane in order to give her a slightly better chance of recovery. They also felt that her unborn baby might have disabilities, despite no medical evidence of this.

Goldie's husband ordered that she be kept alive with a breathing tube. He and her family visited Goldie daily, and she gave birth to a normal child.

Both women emerged from their comas and are on their way to recovery.

Because neither Diane nor Goldie had written instructions on what they wanted done if they could not make decisions, others decided for them. It is important to tell your professionals what *you* want done should *you* be unable to make decisions. Then write it down! Give a copy of your letter to your partner, doctor, lawyer, counselor, and confidant. You'll gain your peace of mind, and possibly your child's life.

CHOOSING AND USING PROFESSIONALS

Every pregnant woman should be under a doctor's care. You may need the assistance of a psychologist, lawyer, social worker, or marriage counselor as well. These professionals should be warm and caring and should treat you and your baby with respect. They should also present a realistic picture of what the future *probably* holds while admitting that there could be a margin of error, no matter how slight. Professionals should respect your intelligence, your right to complete information, and your ability to make your own decisions. Find supportive professionals and lighten your crisis.

"God gives us relatives; thank God, we can choose our friends."

—*Addison Mizner*

Handling Family and Friends

If unsupportive people must eventually know about your pregnancy, plan ahead. Conceal your pregnancy for at least four to six months. Use this book to devise a good plan. Record the plan and your reasons for choosing it in your journal. This saves others the stress of having to plan for you. When you announce your pregnancy, announce your plan. Eventually, your confidence and your ability to view your situation positively will influence those around you.

Use your journal to write a short "pregnancy announcement speech" that reveals your pregnancy and plans. Rehearse the speech in front of a mirror and a confidant. If you must cry or shout, do it in private, not in front of those you wish to tell. Prepare a list of community agencies that are helping you and distribute it during your announcement. Consider asking your confidant and counselor to be on hand during your announcement. Your listeners may restrain extreme emotions when others are present.

Choose a peaceful time to make your announcement, perhaps after a relaxed meal. If anything happens to disrupt the peace, wait for a calmer time. Revealing your crisis during another crisis could create hysteria.

Have your listeners sit down. Ask them to save their questions and comments until you are finished. Then, practicing relaxed breathing to calm yourself (Chapter Two), read your announcement speech from your journal. Your peacefulness will make the anger, disappointment, or anxiety of others seem out of place.

Decide how you'll deal with later blowups. Stick to your plans. If you're pressured, speak to your confidant and to a counselor. They will help you.

Paula and Sheila (mentioned later in this chapter) had well-thought-out plans that helped smooth their pregnancy announcements. So did Adele, whose relatives think that her asthma makes her too weak to mother a large family. Before the last three of her six pregnancies, Adele and her husband had many heart-to-heart talks and found support in two other couples who also had large families. When each pregnancy was getting too obvious, Adele and her husband would tell their families how they had already figured out which room the baby would occupy and how Adele planned to parent another baby.

What is the worst that could happen when you announce your pregnancy? Predict people's responses and decide how to handle them. Preparation is 90 percent of victory!

POOR TIMING

Announcing your pregnancy might bring anything from anger to tears. Decide what to say and do if this happens. Practice remaining calm and in control. If your baby's arrival is poorly timed, remind people that unforeseen circumstances can make any baby's arrival difficult. Let them know that you are reorganizing your plans to include your baby.

Clarissa was worried about renovating a new house after her baby was born, so she and her husband hired a carpenter early in her pregnancy. Renovations were completed the day before Clarissa went into labor.

Clarissa maintains a large garden, does extensive freezing and canning of vegetables, and sells garden produce. Her next baby was due at the beginning of harvest season. Clarissa had her older children help with the housework and let some jobs go undone so that she could breastfeed her baby on demand. By carrying her baby in a backpack carrier, Clarissa kept her hands free to work and survived the summer.

CONCERNS ABOUT IMMATURITY

If people think you're too immature to handle decisions, take control! Your confidence in your plans and your determination to follow them will convince others that you've matured.

Two years before sixteen-year-old Paula's pregnancy, her older teenaged sister's pregnancy shocked her highly respected family and conservative community.

Paula and her boyfriend Ron felt that Paula's parents couldn't cope with another unmarried, pregnant daughter and would never believe that Paula could handle her pregnancy herself.

A PREGNANCY AIDgency volunteer advised Paula to have her baby and promised help. So did Ron's sister, an abortion clinic nurse who liked Paula as a sister. She did not want to see Paula, who was almost four months pregnant, subjected to the trauma of a late abortion. Paula decided to continue attending school and to choose adoption. Her plan eased the shock of her pregnancy announcement, and her family, friends, and community supported her.

DEALING WITH THOSE WHO AVOID YOU

Some individuals may avoid you because you are pregnant. Psychologists call this "fear of contamination," a primitive, subconscious feeling that your pregnancy is "contagious"! No one wants to think that a crisis pregnancy could happen to them, so they avoid you.

You can ask these people, "What is bothering you? Pregnancy isn't contagious." Then include *them* in *your* life. If they still avoid you, let them go. As one true friend told a recovering, formerly suicidal alcoholic, "Remember, a false friend and a shadow stay around only when the sun shines."

CONCERN ABOUT YOUR REPUTATION

If you think that gossip might ruin your reputation, devise a detailed plan and announce your pregnancy before gossip begins. Many highly respected women have withstood gossip, borne their babies, and lived good lives in their communities. Accept yourself and your convictions, and others will accept you, too.

Perhaps you believe that poor moral choices caused your pregnancy. If this is so, admit your error and work on changing your lifestyle. Others will forgive and accept you when they see you are trying to change.

> President of her church youth group and a peer counselor to teens, sixteen-year-old Faila had intercourse once and regretted losing her chastity. As her lover drifted away, Faila denied her pregnancy, then confided in one friend. During a church retreat, Faila came to feel that God would guide her in the right direction if she trusted God's will for her pregnancy. When Faila's mother took her to a doctor because she was concerned that Faila was not menstruating, Faila was in her sixth month of pregnancy.
>
> Faila transferred to a school that had programs for pregnant students. She chose her baby's adoptive parents, had her baby, then returned to her original high school to graduate before going to college. Urging her peers to chastity, Faila again became a youth group leader and peer counselor.

ABUSE AND LOSS OF SHELTER

Could you be abused, verbally or physically, or thrown out of the house because of pregnancy? Before you announce your pregnancy, ask a PREGNANCY AIDgency, women's shelter, or social service agency to have shelter ready. When revealing your pregnancy, have a confidant with you. If your parents abuse you, you can legally be removed from your home. Call a child protection agency or PREGNANCY AIDgency. When sixteen-year-old Sandi's father locked her out of the house because she wouldn't abort, a PREGNANCY AIDgency took her to a shelter home. After Sandi gave birth and decided to parent her baby, her father passed out cigars!

If your baby would be in danger of abuse, ask the abuser to go for counseling. If this person refuses, as is likely to happen, or if counseling is ineffective in stopping the abuse, move into a safer home or a women's shelter. Some women prefer to make adoption plans to protect their children from abuse.

Abused severely and regularly as a child, Clint repeated the pattern and hit his fussing, crying infant son. Clint's wife Jean asked her mother to raise the baby. Jean and Clint visit the baby but leave whenever Clint gets upset.

When Jean became pregnant again, her mother could not raise another child, so Jean and Clint made an adoption plan. The agency keeps them informed about their daughter's progress in her adoptive home. Not wanting to have any more children, Jean chose to be permanently sterilized after her last delivery.

ABUSE FROM A LOVER

If your lover is abusive, consider counseling. A marriage counselor, psychologist, or member of the clergy will help you discover why you continue to love or to live with an abuser. You must understand yourself, evaluate your relationship, and decide whether or not to maintain it.

Occasionally an abuser will consent to counseling, too. Even though this probably won't happen, ask the abuser to seek counseling anyway. If an abuser refuses counseling, it may be best for you to leave. Without outside help, an abuser only gets more violent. Verbal abuse can lead to physical beating. Sometimes abusive relationships end with the death of either the abuser or the abused.

Cycles of Abuse

Abuse can be verbal, physical, or sexual, or all three. Abuse also runs in cycles. Perhaps you are aware of these cycles.

The first phase of the cycle involves several small, abusive incidents that increase in frequency and intensity. This is a tension-building phase in which you try to calm your partner and control the abuse. This phase can end with a severe battering incident, a verbal outburst, or sexual abuse.

After this incident, which in extreme cases may lead to hospitalization, the abuser may enter the loving phase of the cycle. Remorseful, he showers you with love and gifts, promising never to harm you again. However, his promises are empty. With abusers, the first phase of minor abusive incidents probably will begin again.

Mimi planned to have children in five years, after she finished college, but she became pregnant six weeks after marrying Gabe, a serviceman. With her family in another state, Mimi confided her anger and frustration to a consoling friend.

Cool during courtship, Gabe was now cold, distant, and angry. His sexual behavior was bizarre. Eventually, Mimi realized that she had married an alcoholic. When Gabe told Mimi to abort, she refused. He then began to alternate between totally ignoring Mimi and belittling her.

Believing that marriage should be "forever," Mimi clung to prayer, especially to the Bible verse, "All things work together for good for those who love God." When Gabe's inattention to the baby began to turn into physical abuse, Mimi divorced him. A self-help group for relatives of alcoholics gave her support. After years of unemployment and struggle, Mimi now has a career, is finishing her education, and has some firm goals. She is very proud of her daughter.

Can You Make It On Your Own?

You probably have many excuses for staying with an abusive lover. "No one else will love me." "Marriage is forever." "I've got to stay married for the children." "I don't deserve anyone better." "I can't make it on my own." Speak to a counselor. Devise better ways to protect yourself. Consider that men who abuse women often abuse children. Boys who watch abusive fathers often become abusers. Girls who see mothers taking abuse often accept abuse. Even if you are married, you may wish to choose adoption or foster care for your baby.

No one deserves abuse! You and your children have the right to be treated with respect. Call a PREGNANCY AIDgency, a women's resource center, a helpline, or the police for protection. You may have to secretly move somewhere else. While you learn job skills and independent living skills, you can live in a women's shelter or group home. You may have to receive government funds for a while. Eventually, you'll feel capable of living on your own, free of terror.

Linda, an alcoholic and drug addict who was raised in an abusive home, had lost two children to foster care. With no job skills and no self-esteem, she divorced one physically abusive alcoholic and began living with another, who became more abusive when he discovered that Linda was pregnant. Not wanting to raise her child in a violent, alcoholic home, Linda scheduled an abortion.

Feeling ill as she recalled a previous abortion, Linda walked outside the abortion clinic to wait. There she met a woman, a member of a pregnancy counseling group, who allowed Linda to live in her home and continue her pregnancy. By attending alcoholism and drug addiction self-help group meetings, Linda overcame her addictions and learned to refuse abuse. Once she called the police to arrest her boyfriend; another time she obtained a restraining order against him.

Linda obtained visitation rights with her other children. The woman with whom she stayed, and others, taught Linda some job skills. Today, government assistance pays for Linda's small apartment as Linda parents her baby. She hopes to get a job when her baby is older.

PRESSURE FROM OTHERS TO ABORT

You will lessen outside pressure on you to abort by waiting as long as possible before announcing your pregnancy. Many people believe that abortion late in pregnancy is illegal. This may not be true, but if it helps to keep unwanted advisors at a distance, don't tell them!

In many areas, abortion is legal until birth. Don't assume that no one will perform an abortion on you if you are six or seven or eight months pregnant. If you are a teen and you fear that your parents will pressure you to abort, you may be eligible for a court-appointed guardian. If your husband or lover pressures you, you may choose to live elsewhere. A lawyer, PREGNANCY AIDgency, or social service agency for women or children can help you.

If you are forcefully taken to an abortion clinic, tell the personnel that you are being forced to have an abortion. State that you will sue the clinic if they perform the abortion against your will. Do not allow anyone to drag you anywhere or give you any medication. Do not sign anything. Scream if necessary. Not wanting to perform an abortion against your will, the clinic will probably send you home, where the pressure will continue. If you don't want to cave in, *call your local PREGNANCY AIDgency immediately. They definitely can help you!*

> *Although fifteen-year-old Sheila wanted to have her baby, her parents insisted that she abort. Secretly, Sheila contacted a PREGNANCY AIDgency volunteer counselor who took her to a lawyer.*
>
> *Her lawyer advised her of her options. Because she was pregnant, she could receive medical aid. She could place a restraining order on her parents so that they could no longer mentally harass her. Then, either the PREGNANCY AIDgency or the lawyer would have custody of Sheila and become her legal guardian. She would no longer need parental consent to be sheltered in a private home. If she decided against filing a restraining order, her parents might possibly take her to an abortion clinic against her wishes. If this were to happen, the lawyer said, Sheila should then instruct both the nurses and the abortionist that she did not want an abortion. She should not sign any clinic forms and should tell the abortionist that she would sue when she became of legal age if an abortion was performed.*
>
> *Sheila and a PREGNANCY AIDgency volunteer confronted her parents with the two options. Sheila's parents conceded and allowed her to move into a shelter home. Ultimately, they relented and allowed Sheila to parent her baby. They grew to be doting grandparents.*

GROUP PRESSURE

You may be part of a group that will disapprove of your having your baby. Even if you hide your pregnancy for a long time, the group is going to find out about it eventually, unless you decide to keep your pregnancy a secret forever, as discussed in Chapter Two. However, you may feel a certain hypocrisy in staying with a group that would shun you if they knew you gave birth. You may have to decide if you want to remain with this group.

Some groups that might pressure you about your pregnancy are sororities, religious groups, clubs, or professional groups whose members shun, gossip about, or ignore those who do not conform. Other groups that may exert pressure include feminist, environmental, or population control groups that believe children should be planned and family size should be limited. Pressure to abort the child you didn't plan on having can be subtle and powerful, even if never actually voiced. Group members who favor abortion may expect you to "correct your mistake." You may have mixed feelings about your group, since you admire its goals and philosophies yet dislike the pressure to conform to a rigid code of behavior.

Other groups are more blatant in their ability to control their members. These include personality-dominated groups whose dynamic, charismatic leaders promote certain philosophies, religions, or lifestyles. Some of these groups are cults and gangs. These groups often control members by using violence, threats, and harassment. You may hear that the time is not right for you to give birth, and that dire consequences may take place if you do.

Be suspicious of any person or group that tries to manipulate you with fear, humiliation, degradation, or conformity. You will find it difficult to evaluate group dynamics by yourself. You may need help from a trained counselor to decide what is best for you and your baby.

Discuss the questions in Appendix F with a counselor, psychologist, or member of the clergy and learn how to feel confident making your own decisions. A PREGNANCY AIDgency can help you with your pregnancy.

You may decide that your group has admirable goals. Even if its members believe in pregnancy planning, the baby you didn't plan on having can learn from you to make the world better. Or, if you can't parent, you can help influence your child by choosing an adoptive family whose views are similar to yours. Parented well, your child may come to advance your group's cause in ways you cannot yet possibly imagine.

Tell your group how you feel about having your baby and why. If your ideas have changed, admit it. Look for a supportive group member. If your group cannot accept your pregnancy, you may prefer to join a similar, more supportive group or to start your own group.

An active feminist, Joyce endured one pregnancy she didn't plan, convinced that women shouldn't have to bear babies they didn't want. Pregnant again at forty, Joyce had three children in school and needed to work to pay off debts. She went to three doctors in three states to get an abortion. Each said that her reasons for wanting an abortion weren't good enough, so she glumly endured her pregnancy. By the time her son was born, she very much wanted him.

Joyce began to work for abortion rights, but she said that her research slowly convinced her that feminism must include both the mother and the unborn child. Leaving her abortion rights group, Joyce began to speak and write about her own views.

Joyce's first, planned daughter loves her mother, but because she lives in another state, she sees Joyce only occasionally. The daughter she didn't plan on having lives nearby and visits Joyce frequently. Joyce's planned son was brutally murdered. Caring for the son she didn't plan helped Joyce to overcome her grief. Joyce acknowledges that the children she didn't plan to have brought her much joy. "God has a plan for pregnancy surprises," she says.

You may decide that the group you belong to or the person you are following is too strange, untrustworthy, or even dangerous. You may decide to part company. If so, you might need help over a long period of time, including psychological counseling, life management skills, treatment for addictions, police protection, and medication. However, you *can* make a new future for yourself and for your baby. Believe in what you can do!

Regina, a popular, straight-A student, tried to convert Satanist students at her school to Christianity, but, instead, she converted to Satanism. Physically abused and raped at a Satanic party, she became pregnant. A counseling agency that assists victims of Satanism helped her release her fears about the personality of her baby. She has decided to give birth and is seeing a psychologist to help her regain her self-respect, faith, and goals.

WHEN YOUR PARTNER DOESN'T WANT A BABY

Has your partner threatened to leave if you get pregnant? You may not really have to choose between your lover and your baby. See if he fits into one of the categories that follow. If he does, you may be able to calm his fears or reassure him.

- The **insecure lover** has many fears: Will a baby rob him of your love? Will pregnancy make you press for marriage? How will he ever be a good father?

    What are your partner's fears? To find out, start a conversation with him about someone's pregnancy or baby. Listen to your partner's comments. Try to understand his fears, then calm them.

    Lavish him with love and assure him that you love him more than ever. If he's afraid you'll press for marriage, say that marriage is not on your mind. Emphasize his positive, loving traits and help him understand how he can be a good dad. Or make an adoption plan. If you calm his fears, the insecure lover will often accept his baby.

- The **misinformed lover** thinks it's best for you not to have a baby now.

    Show the misinformed lover this book. Assure him that you want to have your baby and that you have plans under way to do so. If you educate him about the support available for pregnant women, he will probably support you.

- The **child-shy man** doesn't like children and doesn't want to be a father. Ever. No matter what you do, he may remain firm. If you would rather have a relationship with him than with your baby, consider adoption.

    However, the child-shy man may become the doting father once he realizes what the baby kicking around in your womb means to him. Get the child-shy man into a doctor's office by telling him that you have a serious problem (don't say what). Before the visit, arrange to have the doctor let this man hear his baby's heartbeat on a fetal heart monitor or view his baby on a sonogram. Hearing or seeing the baby may soften him.

- The **abusive, manipulative lover** sees women as bodies to be used and sometimes abused. He may physically or verbally pressure you to abort, and may leave you if you don't. An earlier discussion in this chapter may help you decide if you want to stay with this man.

WHEN YOU OR OTHERS REJECT YOUR CHILD

You may feel you don't want your baby. Perhaps your child is not the sex you desired. Maybe you conceived the child with a man you don't love. You may hate the circumstances surrounding the pregnancy. If you can't overcome your rejection, repulsion, or disappointment, consider making an adoption plan. But give yourself time. Your feelings may change as birth draws close.

Even though *others* may reject your child, you can parent your child if *your* love is strong enough. Your love may slowly erode the rejection of your baby by others. This is what happened to Sandi and Sheila (mentioned earlier in this chapter).

The Biracial Child

If you're pregnant with a biracial child, you may have a hard time accepting your baby. Others may reject your biracial baby as well. You could reject your baby if you are pregnant after being raped by a man of a different race. Or, you may have loved your baby's father once but did not consider racial mix important until your relationship started to crumble. Now you may hate the man you once loved. Even if you and your lover are still together, prejudiced family members or friends may view a biracial love affair as "wrong" or "foolish," and they may not accept your baby.

How do you feel about your baby's racial mix? Do you hate your baby's father or harbor deep-seated prejudices against his race? If speaking to a counselor doesn't dispel your hatred and prejudice, consider making an adoption plan for your baby.

Do you love your baby's father or feel attraction or indifference toward members of his race? You'll probably love and accept his child. If your biracial child resulted from an affair, refer to information later in this chapter for guidance.

If others are prejudiced, remind them that all races are of equal value. Race has nothing to do with your child's worth or your motherly love.

If prejudiced talk continues, say, "Excuse me, but I prefer not to listen to this," and then politely leave.

Many children, like single mom Roxanna's biracial daughter (Chapter Two) and Fran's biracial son (later in this chapter), live in communities and attend schools with many biracial children. These children rarely experience stigma. Other children aren't so lucky. If your child would experience social stigma in your area, consider making an adoption plan for your baby or moving to another area.

A white woman living in a small, bigoted community, Shannie bore a biracial child after two men, one white and one black, raped her. Shunned and laughed at by the community, Shannie and her son were treated as outcasts. Shannie worked as a seamstress and received government assistance. She hated her poverty and despaired about her son's future.

When the boy was three years old, a national newspaper story made public Shannie's plight. A prominent business person set up a trust fund for Shannie's son. Using some of this money, Shannie moved to a large city where she made a down payment on a small house and secured a good job. Growing up among other biracial children, her son is proud of who he is and is doing very well in school. Shannie receives counseling to resolve the anger that she still experiences because of the sexual assault.

If you live in a prejudiced community, you'll have to build your child's self-esteem. Books can give you ideas to help your child feel capable, hopeful, worthwhile, and self-confident.

FEELING GOOD ABOUT TELLING OTHERS THAT YOU'RE PREGNANT

Handling family and friends will require tact, confidence, and a detailed plan. Devise ways to deal with upsetting reactions before they occur. Planning will increase the chance of a positive response. Think positively, avoid negative thinkers, and manage stress. Most people who react dramatically at first will eventually accept your decisions. You needed time to adjust to your pregnancy. They will need time, too.

"Only the wise know how to love."

—*Seneca*

Influencing Your Love Relationships

How nice it would be if every baby were born into a loving, supportive relationship! But life is not ideal. Often, we must work with what is, rather than what we think should be. To do this, you must first examine the complications and emotions involved in your love relationship. Then you can plan for your baby.

IF YOU ARE UNMARRIED

Being unmarried and pregnant doesn't bring the stigma or rejection that it used to. Some unmarried women purposely become pregnant. If your family and boyfriend would support you in your pregnancy, your biggest problem may be that your sexual relationship or pregnancy is about to become public knowledge. Embarrassment is not fatal! You should be able to plan successfully for the future.

Because sixteen-year-old Julie's parents promoted chastity among teens, Julie's pregnancy was a terrible crisis. Surviving gossip, financial setback, and embarrassment, the family helped parent Julie's daughter until Julie graduated from college, began a career, and married the child's father.

Julie's boyfriend stuck by her. Will yours stick by you? He may be using you by promising marriage but never following through. Give your lover an ultimatum—

have him either make a commitment to you or leave. Be firm. You need to know how he fits into your life.

> *By setting a marriage date, Nathan persuaded Sally to have intercourse one night when she had been drinking. Although she felt used, Sally wanted marriage and soon was having sex frequently. She became pregnant. Throughout her pregnancy, Nathan kept postponing the marriage date until Sally's uncle told him, "Either marry Sally now, or get out of her life." Nathan left. Sally, who had been living with distant relatives to keep her pregnancy a secret, made an adoption plan. Nathan's mother called, promising Nathan would marry her if she'd parent the baby. "Let Nathan call himself," Sally said. He didn't. After completing the adoption, Sally returned to college.*

AFFAIRS AND PREGNANCY

A love affair complicates your life. Really! Whether you're the other woman or you have two lovers, you've been walking a tightrope. Why did you enter into an affair? What will you do now? A member of the clergy or a marriage counselor can help you evaluate an affair and understand your motives. A social service agency may be able to arrange affordable counseling. You need to answer questions such as those in Appendix F.

If your lover is tolerant, he may suspect or know about the affair but not care. Maybe you don't care if he has other lovers. Evaluate your lifestyle. Maybe it's time for a change or a commitment.

If one or both lovers are jealous, you'll be afraid to let them know about each other. One lover might even become violent toward you or toward the other man. You'll have to know how to protect yourself and your baby in addition to deciding which of the relationships, if any, you want to preserve.

Before ending a relationship, hold your lover to any promises he's made. Give him an ultimatum: if he's married, he must file within one month for divorce. If he's single, he must say good-bye to any other lovers. Give him another month to "set the date," preferably for marriage to you. If, within two months, a lover cannot break any other relationships and be committed to you alone, he will never do it.

If your lover offered you only false promises, decide what you will do. If you end one relationship, end it quickly. Tell your lover you'll no longer see him, and then do it.

Who's the Baby's Father?

You may know, or think you know, who your baby's father is. Ask yourself, "Could the man I'm planning to stay with be my baby's father?" He could be if you are having sexual relations with him, even if you are doing so only occasionally. He could be the father even if he has had a vasectomy or has a fertility problem. Only medical testing can prove otherwise. This subject will be discussed in further detail later in this chapter.

The man whom you are planning to stay with will probably assume the baby is his unless you tell him otherwise. If there is no way the baby could be his, you will have to either hide your pregnancy, fabricate a story about how it happened, or admit to having had an affair.

Who will the baby look like? The lover you're leaving? Will everyone suspect your baby's true father? Not unless you tell about your affair.

You have blood relatives. So does the man whom you've chosen to stay with. Decide which one of these relatives looks somewhat like the man you think is your baby's actual father. If anyone remarks about your baby's appearance, comment that your child certainly does bear a strong resemblance to that particular relative.

Both married to others, Peg and Hal concealed a fifteen-year affair, which resulted in a son whom Peg raised along with the children of her marriage. Only when the boy was nine, and Hal's wife discovered Peg's photo in Hal's wallet, did the truth come out. Peg's husband wished to grant Peg a divorce to marry Hal, but Hal's wife refused to divorce Hal. Peg realized that she should have chosen between the two men long ago.

Revealing Your Affair

Should you disclose your affair? Who knows about it already? Who will benefit if you do get it out in the open? If you need help dealing with your feelings and don't know what to do, speak to a counselor. Remember that you can talk to one freely and be assured of confidentiality.

You may feel that your partner deserves the truth. Perhaps someone suspects the affair, or you and your partner have not been having intercourse, or your baby was fathered by a man of another race. If you don't want to claim that you're pregnant from rape, and you don't want to live elsewhere until after the baby is born, you may want to tell about your affair before it becomes common knowledge.

Admitting that you've had an affair can be frightening. Tell a family counselor or member of the clergy about your situation and predict your partner's reaction. Telling your partner in the presence of this counselor will ease the shock. Both you and your partner may need several counseling sessions before you can begin to make plans for the baby. Through a counselor, Pearl and Ken (Chapter Five) made an adoption plan for a baby conceived during an affair.

If you wish to parent your child, your partner will have to sort through his feelings for the baby. Perhaps he can accept and love this child as his own.

After a troubled youth, Fran married Peter, a very understanding man. Following the birth of her third child, Fran had a love affair with Dean, a man of another race. Pregnant with Dean's child, Fran knew that her husband would love and forgive her, and told him of her affair with Dean.

Peter accepts and loves as his own this biracial child. If someone asks where Fran adopted her son, she responds, "He's mine," and refuses to discuss the details, since she doesn't "have to explain another person's reason for being." When her son gets older, she plans to tell him the truth about his conception.

If you prefer to go somewhere else to give birth, and then convince your husband that you've adopted someone else's baby, refer to Chapter Two.

SURVIVING PREGNANCY IN A BROKEN LOVE RELATIONSHIP

Are you facing divorce, separation, widowhood, or the breakup of a relationship? What emotions are you feeling? What is causing these feelings?

If your husband or lover died, the pain of loss might be unbearable. Reach beyond grieving family and friends for guidance. A counselor, member of the clergy, or support group for the bereaved will help you to understand your emotions and to gather enough strength to plan for your baby.

When Kimberly's husband died in a tragic accident, she was left with one child and pregnant with twins. Shock, anger, and rejection of her babies yielded to love for her children and a determination to succeed in life. Inspiring books, songs, and movies, in addition to time, slowly helped to lift the depression of widowhood and the strain of living with overbearing relatives.

When the twins were four, Kimberly moved away and completed high school and college, earning two degrees. Today her children are grown, and Kimberly is a highly respected writer, lecturer, and television producer.

Divorce or breakup can cause confusion. Perhaps your lover left you, possibly for another woman. Or perhaps you ended the relationship. You might be angry at yourself, your lover, and your baby. People may misunderstand the situation or offer poor advice. A trained counselor will help you deal with your emotions and make plans. Divorced and about to begin a high-paying job, Evaleen was pressured by her family to abort. Her ex-husband advised her to give birth. With a PREG-NANCY AIDgency's guidance, Evaleen has continued her career while parenting her son, who has, she said, "fulfilled my life."

What Changes Will Have to Be Made?

When a love relationship ends, you will have to cope with life without your mate. A counselor can help you understand what adjustments will have to be made. These might include finding a place to live and furniture, obtaining custody of your children or visitation rights, or acquiring job skills and a job. You may need to learn living skills such as budgeting, car maintenance, house upkeep, or single parenting. Legal, financial, medical, or real estate advice may help you. You may need to sort through your lover's belongings and dispose of them. You probably also need time to yourself, and someone to talk to about the grief, anger, or pain you're feeling. Defining and meeting your own needs will clear up some confusion and help you make better plans for your baby.

How do you feel about your baby? Do you resent or pity this child? Or do you see this baby as your lover's final gift? No matter how you feel now, you may deeply love your child in time. You may want to parent. Work through your emotions, make plans for your baby, and keep your options open.

After just about everyone—relatives, friends, and social worker alike—told Shelley to abort, she found encouragement in one of her sisters and decided to give birth. Since her partner Frank was immature, hypocritical, and irresponsible, Shelley considered making an adoption plan for her baby, but decided to break up with Frank and be a single parent.

Knowing that he was a father, Frank obtained a job and settled down. He and Shelley married just days before their baby was born. They now have two children and are a very happy family.

THE VASECTOMY ALIBI

If your partner had a vasectomy and you've been loyal to him and still got pregnant, then either the vasectomy was unsuccessful or you had intercourse too soon after the vasectomy was performed. A doctor can examine your lover and discover what happened. As you get over your initial shock, you can plan for the baby. A sense of humor and a great deal of love definitely help!

Everyone knew that Vera's husband Jim had a vasectomy during his previous marriage. However, two months after the wedding, Vera was pregnant!

Delighted to be a father, Jim wanted more children. Vera was glad about her pregnancy, too, but embarrassed because, she said, "People will think that I'm running around with someone else."

"Nobody's going to think that," Jim said jokingly, shaking his fist.

Although Vera wondered if people gossiped about her pregnancy, no one made any direct remarks. Vera had a daughter. During the fourth month of her second pregnancy, doctors discovered uterine cancer, so Vera had a hysterectomy following her son's birth.

Vera laughs about how her "sterile" husband fathered two children. She wonders how many children she would have had if she had not had a hysterectomy.

Vera's husband actually had a vasectomy, but it was unsuccessful. Your lover, however, may have lied to you. By claiming to have had a vasectomy, some men might more easily persuade women to have sexual relationships. If you suspect that your partner lied, confront him. In the first three months after a vasectomy, only 1 out of 200 vasectomies is unsuccessful. After three months, only 1 out of 2,000 vasectomies fails. Vasectomy failure rate is very low.

Don't assume that your partner will sheepishly tell you the truth. He may insist that he actually had a vasectomy. Ask which doctor performed the vasectomy, and when and where it was performed. If your lover can't come up with this information, your suspicions may be true. If he does give you names and places, he should be willing to have the doctor assure you that the operation was performed.

If a man lied to you about a vasectomy, he has probably told other lies, too. Consider breaking off a relationship with a man you can't trust. Then decide what to do about your baby.

Some men who claim to have had vasectomies accuse their pregnant lovers of being unfaithful. If you have been faithful, suggest that a doctor examine your lover to determine if the vasectomy was unsuccessful. A man who refuses to submit to an exam is probably lying about his vasectomy or else he's so overbearing that he refuses an examination because *you* suggested it. Some men prefer self-righteous jealousy to the truth. Do you want a relationship with this type of person?

Suppose your lover did have a vasectomy, but you have been unfaithful. Earlier sections of this chapter and the questions in Appendix F will help you think more clearly about your affair and your pregnancy.

IF ONE OF YOU HAS A FERTILITY PROBLEM

You or your partner may have a fertility problem. Doctors may have told you that you would never be able to give birth. Now that you have become comfortable with your childless lifestyle, your pregnancy has caught you off guard.

Most couples who were previously infertile adjust quickly to having a baby. Guidelines in this book can help you adjust, too. Many couples parent their children. Others make adoption plans for their babies.

If your partner has a fertility problem and you're pregnant, you may find yourself wondering if others will think that you became pregnant as a result of an affair. If you didn't, try to be like Vera (earlier in this chapter) and Barb (Chapter Four) by developing a sense of humor. Although it took two years of artificial insemination with her husband's sperm before Barb became pregnant the first time, a few years later she became pregnant unexpectedly. Despite the constant nausea she felt with both of her pregnancies, and the threat of miscarriage that she experienced with each, Barb was delighted to give birth to both of her babies.

LOVING IN SPITE OF THE PAIN

Some love relationships complicate pregnancy. You have difficult choices and adjustments to make in some confusing situations. Simplify things by smoothing out your love life. Then, plan for your baby. A counselor or confidant can help you and your lover define problems and make plans.

No matter what your love relationships are, don't overlook another relationship—that is, the love that you should feel for yourself and for your baby. Do you love yourself and your child? If you don't, seek counseling. When you love yourself, you can more easily handle other love difficulties. Then the decisions you make will be best for both you and your baby.

> *"Remember this also, and be well persuaded of its truth:*
> *the future is not in the hands of Fate, but in ours."*
>
> —Jules Jusserand

Continuing Your Education and Career

Continuing an education or advancing a career may help you have the life you desire. Can you have your baby without giving up your future plans? Certainly!

EDUCATION

If you're in high school, vocational school, or college, you may be considering dropping out of school or college, at least for a while, to parent. Education is valuable. Even if you have to go to school part-time for a while, it may be wiser to continue with your education while you parent.

Women who drop out of school often regret their choice and have great difficulty motivating themselves to go back to school and complete their education. Moreover, they may resent their children for "causing" them to sacrifice their education. Before you fall into this trap, answer the questions in Appendix F, read this section, and discuss your options with a confidant and an educational counselor. This pregnancy won't ruin your education. Many pregnant women, both married and single, complete their education. You can, too.

If you're threatened with expulsion from your school, contact a lawyer. In most situations, it is illegal to expel you from school or college for pregnancy. Even a private institution may be brought up on charges if it discriminates against a pregnant woman. A lawyer can advise you.

Speak to a school or college counselor or nurse about your pregnancy and any adjustments you must make with regard to classes. If a nurse or counselor pressures you to abort, speak to an administrator. Educational employees should support you, not badger you. If the pressure gets severe, ask a PREGNANCY AIDgency to contact the administration, or threaten to take your story to the local newspaper. Either of these actions will probably end the pressure.

Cope with discomforts. Catnap in the nurse's office if you tire easily. Carry low-salt crackers in your purse and munch on them to fight nausea. Walking to class is good exercise and releases stress. Ask for different desks if seating becomes awkward.

Your doctor can arrange for adjustments in physical education classes or sports. If you're trying to hide your pregnancy, have a PREGNANCY AIDgency ask your physical education instructor, coach, and guidance counselor to keep your secret. Tell your classmates whatever you like to explain your altered gym or sports routine. If you're afraid the institution would reveal your secret, tell a PREGNANCY AIDgency. You may be able to relocate to another school or college, have a doctor sign an excuse for you (without mentioning pregnancy), or make another plan.

Classmates will adjust to your pregnancy. If any of them pressure you to abort, remember that many students and faculty have had abortions or have supported those who did. Be firm in your decision to give birth, and others will soon support you. If you're single, your community may take longer than your classmates to accept your pregnancy, but it will do so in time. Despite her pregnancy, popular, congenial Jill was elected senior prom queen over the objections of some community members. After graduating with honors and giving birth to a son, Jill married her fiancé.

Alternatives

If you want to continue your education, but not at your school or college, request a home tutor. If your request is denied, a PREGNANCY AIDgency may be able to locate a tutor. Ask about taking courses with a home study option. Mail in course work and keep up with your classes. You may want to skip a semester and return to class after giving birth, or take classes at another institution where no one knows you. Be sure that you can transfer your credits to your original school or college.

What plans will you make for your baby while you are attending school? If you decide to parent, you may want to take some time off from school until the baby is a few months old. Perhaps you'll just keep going to class. Some large high schools and college campuses have day-care centers for students' children. If yours doesn't, perhaps a friend or relative, day-care center, or baby sitter can care for your baby while you're in class. If you'll graduate soon, foster care may care temporarily for your baby. Sixteen when she became pregnant, Julie (mentioned earlier in this chapter) completed high school while her parents watched her baby. Wendy, also sixteen when she became pregnant, lived with her boyfriend and went on welfare when he joined the United States Navy. An A student, Wendy used in-school day care for her child while she completed her education.

You may have to lobby to have family housing facilities at your college campus opened to single mothers. If the college refuses, ask the college to house you in an apartment for the same fee you'd pay for on-campus family housing. If the college still refuses, tell the administration that you will speak to the press, a lawyer, or a civil liberties union, and then do so. Single-parent families have a right to family housing.

A graduate student, Felice decided to stop feeling guilty about her pregnancy, and severed ties with her unemployed, unstable, threatening boyfriend. She continued to take courses and earn money as a college assistant.

The public health system paid for her medical care. A social service agency gave Felice information on child care and referred her to a support group for pregnant women. After Felice requested an apartment in married student housing, the housing opened up to single mothers and is called ''family housing'' today. After her baby's birth, Felice continued as a graduate assistant and took independent study classes. She and other mothers took turns babysitting for each other's children.

If you want to continue your education, you may wish to choose adoption so that you will have more freedom, or, if you are single, so that your child will have the benefit of two parents. Chapter Five discusses adoption in detail.

CAREER

As a career woman, you're used to managing your life. You may feel stupid or careless for becoming pregnant. Will coworkers consider you unenlightened if you have your baby? Not if you're firm about it. You have several options available. You may choose adoption, decide to stay home with your baby, or combine your career with motherhood.

Married and single career women in very public positions are having babies. Confidently announce your plans and expect acceptance. A well-known, unmarried anchorwoman on a large television station, Esther went public with the pregnancy she didn't plan, and continued her career as a single mother. Yolanda and her husband (Chapter One) have chosen their careers over parenting by placing their two children in adoptive homes. Aimee and her husband made an adoption plan for their first child so that they could successfully launch their careers and become financially secure. They plan to have more children and parent them later on.

If your employer threatens to fire you because you're pregnant, contact a PREGNANCY AIDgency, women's resource center, lawyer, or civil liberties union. Although employers can move you to a different job or take safety precautions, they probably cannot legally fire you just because you're pregnant. You may have grounds for a lawsuit.

You may work throughout your pregnancy or take maternity leave. If you prefer to leave your job temporarily, request a specific leave of absence. You may prefer to find a new job.

You can choose from a vast network of child care services to use when you go back to work, including day care, live-in nanny, babysitting, nursery school, and preschool. You can hire a housekeeper or employ a housecleaning service. Your greatest crisis may be deciding when and if to return to your career, and you face the chore of finding good child care when you do. Questions in Appendix F may help you make good decisions.

Some mothers find that they can remain at home and still work for pay. Jobs that can be performed in the home include the grooming of pets, the teaching of health fitness courses, and cottage industries such as the making and selling of crafts or foods. For a listing of over 200 ways to make money by working from your home, write to Focus on the Family, Pomona, California 91799, and request that group's fact sheet on cottage industries.

Military Career

A soldier in the United States Army, Alice has never been married and is the mother of two girls. She lives in rent-free, on-base housing and utilizes the base day-care center while on duty.

You, too, can combine a military career with motherhood. Whether you are married or single, you probably cannot be discharged from the military because you're pregnant. If you are threatened with discharge, contact a lawyer or PREGNANCY AIDgency. You should also discuss any potentially hazardous working conditions with your commanding officer and request a transfer if you or your baby could be exposed to radiation, harmful chemicals, or other hazards.

Physically Demanding Careers

If you're in a physically demanding career such as sports or dance, you may fear that your pregnancy will get you out of condition. Mary Decker Slaney, Valerie Brisco, and Evelyn Ashford are three track stars who have successfully combined motherhood with a sports career. Each has participated in the Olympics and won several medals. Many other mothers are in physically demanding careers, too. If you're in top physical condition, ask your doctor if you can continue your current physical activity until your sixth month of pregnancy or beyond. Whenever you exercise, protect your baby by keeping your body temperature below 101°F, and follow any other guidelines a doctor gives you. As your pregnancy progresses, you may prefer doing less strenuous exercises and drills, and then easing back into shape after your baby's birth. By the same time next year, you should be in top condition again.

When Nadine, a professional ballet dancer, married and became pregnant, she stopped dancing professionally but continued to take classes until her fifth month of pregnancy. When her baby was a few months old, she returned to classes and did extensive exercises so that she could dance in the Christmas ballet The Nutcracker.

Keeping Your Pregnancy a Secret at Work

If you don't want anyone to know you're pregnant, follow the suggestions in Chapter Two. If you're the owner, manager, or executive of a business or corporation, formulate a reason for going away for a few months. Then begin to look for a temporary replacement. By maintaining contact by phone, your establishment can survive in your absence.

If you're an employee, you'll need to take time off without threat of losing your job. Will a certain boss keep your secret and hold your job? Might your boss be more sympathetic if a PREGNANCY AIDgency makes the contact?

If you don't feel comfortable with any supervisor and you don't want to change jobs, try making yourself an "indispensable" worker. Be self-assured and reliable: care about your job and work diligently. Then request a few months leave of absence, beginning around the time you feel you can no longer conceal your pregnancy. Say that you need to care for a relative, work out some personal matters, or do whatever else seems plausible. Ask your employer to hold your job, and volunteer to help find a temporary replacement. Offer to do some work from your temporary location. If all goes well, your employer will grant you a leave of absence and your job will be secure.

If you have trouble getting a leave of absence, ask a PREGNANCY AIDgency to speak in your favor, perhaps without revealing your pregnancy. If this fails, work as long as possible, move into a PREGNANCY AIDgency shelter, and prepare some resumés. You'll be able to find another job after your baby is born. Meanwhile, unemployment compensation should help you.

Balancing your pregnancy with an education or career requires adjustments. Some of these will be minor, others major. With the help of your confidant, PREGNANCY AIDgency volunteer, or counselor, you will be able to make the adjustments with the least amount of stress. Problems work themselves out in time. Soon your pregnancy will fit into your new lifestyle.

"You can put a body in prison, but the soul has wings."

—M.P.N.

Handling Pregnancy in Prison

Today more women than ever are being put in prison, and more of them are pregnant when they enter. You might be a hardened criminal, a naive prostitute, a teen-aged shoplifter, or a drug user. Being pregnant and in prison can be frightening. You're worried about your baby and yourself.

A few prisons and county jails are sensitive to the medical and emotional needs of pregnant women. In these, you'll receive excellent care. You may even be able to parent your baby in these prisons.

However, many prisons neglect the special needs of pregnant women. If you ask to see a doctor, request prenatal vitamins, or complain of illness or pain, you may be ignored or given medications that are unsafe for your unborn child. Because you're pregnant, you need to eat a high-protein and high-fiber diet, but you probably won't get it in prison. Your cell mates might have contagious illnesses. You may have to go off alcohol or drugs "cold turkey," which could be dangerous to your baby. You probably won't receive much prenatal care.

After you give birth, or if you miscarry, the prison staff might be insensitive to any postpartum depression or physical problems that you might suffer. Shortly after birth, your baby will probably be taken away. If you don't arrange for parenting, your child may go into foster care and then be adopted, even without your consent.

ADVOCATES

There are people who will help you in any way they can while you are pregnant and in prison. Because they act on your behalf, they are called advocates. Contact a group that will act as advocate for you, or have a friend or relative contact a group. You're fortunate if you have a prison advocacy group nearby. It will provide you with the help you need. Your second best choice is a PREGNANCY AIDgency. Most PREGNANCY AIDgencies will accept collect phone calls. You may have no money to make a long distance phone call to another agency that will not accept collect calls, and the prison will probably not pay for your calls. Ask a PREGNANCY AIDgency to call other agencies for you. You might also contact a women's resource center, a civil liberties union, or a church's social justice committee. Any of these groups may be able to provide advocates who will help you and your unborn child.

Your advocates will speak to prison officials, local groups, and national prisoner advocacy groups (see Appendix H) to get specific help for you.

Advocates should attempt to have you receive a shorter or changed sentence because you are pregnant. Or they might request an alternative to imprisonment. If you must stay in prison, advocates may be able to arrange for medical care, prenatal vitamins, childbirth classes, and postnatal care, and to pay for these services and dietary supplements if the prison refuses to do so.

If you're promised a shorter sentence or other favors if you abort your baby, your advocates should support you in your decision to give birth. If they don't, then they aren't helping you, and you should select different advocates. If the pressure to abort gets extreme, contact a lawyer, a pro-life group, or a civil liberties union. Prison officials cannot force you to have an abortion and cannot legally make life miserable for you if you don't have one. A lawyer can handle this situation. Contact a PREGNANCY AIDgency or prisoners' advocacy group if you are unable to pay for legal advice.

PARENTING YOUR BABY

Being in prison doesn't mean that you are automatically a poor parent. It does mean that you have some real problems to solve. It's unfair to raise your child when you get out of prison if you could face another arrest. You may have to learn skills, change attitudes, or make new friends in order to keep "clean" after you are released. Join a self-help anonymous group, a women's group, or a religious group, or attend sessions arranged through a mental health or social service agency. Group members can help you learn ways to deal with pressure.

If you plan on parenting your baby after you get out of prison, advocates will be able to help you find someone to parent your baby in a safe environment while you're in prison. A partner, relative, friend, or foster family may do this. Your advocate should try to have you parent your baby as long as possible and should also work for frequent visitation with your children and partner, visitation that allows physical contact. If you are planning to marry, advocates can make arrangements.

Advocates can find people to teach you skills in parenting, discipline, housekeeping, and meal planning, as well as job skills. You may need new housing or you may want to relocate to escape your past. Perhaps you will need legal advice, religious guidance, or marital, family, or psychological counseling.

If you choose to make an adoption plan for your baby, you can straighten out your life while giving your baby a stable home. Advocates can bring you and an adoption agency together. Perhaps the prison will allow you to make the type of adoption plan you want.

If you're still in contact with your partner, he and any children you have will have to know about your baby, especially if you're planning to parent the baby yourself. If they can't visit you often, write letters to them, or have an advocate write the letters for you. Some prisons may allow you to tape-record your messages and mail them home.

YOU AS ADVOCATE

Getting help in prison may require that you change your personality and the way you are used to getting things done. You may be used to bullying your way into power, demanding change, or taking what you want. When working with prison officials, gentle and kind persistence is more likely to get you what you need.

Prison officials see themselves as authorities who deserve respect. The saying "You can catch more flies with honey than with vinegar" definitely holds true when requesting help from prison officials. Be polite and cooperative, yet persistent. Avoid the image of troublemaker. When you do receive help, even the most basic help, generously thank those who gave it. You'll be more likely to receive help again.

Help prison officials to understand how helping *you* will actually help *them*. Show that your requests will make *less* work, not more. Dale Carnegie's classic book *How to Win Friends and Influence People* offers excellent advice on working with those who may be unsympathetic to your cause. Be patient. You may not get all that you request, but you should get some help.

> *Drug abusers Pam and Molly were both carrying high-risk pregnancies, yet received little prenatal care in prison without lobbying for it.*
>
> *For a time, Pam lived in maximum security in a poorly lighted, barren, and shabby cell. She got little exercise and was shackled whenever she left the prison grounds. Her back pains went untreated until she actively confronted the health services unit. Having lost four children when her mother obtained custody of them and moved away, Pam bore two more in prison. Her father and stepsister care for one child, and a prisoners' advocacy group found a local family to care for the other. The couple often brings the baby to see Pam.*
>
> *Molly's family arranged for an early release date if she'd enroll in a substance abuse clinic and also take a psychologist's advice to abort. Rachel and Victoria, jailed briefly after an abortion clinic protest, supported Molly's decision to give birth and tried to get her prenatal vitamins, care, and treatment for her asthma. They were unsuccessful until Molly was seventeen weeks pregnant, two weeks before her release date. After a short stay in a shelter for pregnant women, Molly lived with Victoria and received medical assistance, food stamps, and help from a PREGNANCY AIDgency. She avoided drugs and alcohol and even quit smoking! When her son was a few weeks old, she moved into a girlfriend's apartment. With Victoria's and Rachel's help, she is trying to make a new life.*

A NEW LIFE

You can have a new life, too. Prison can hold your body, but not your soul. If you want to be free of the past and make a future for yourself and your baby, you can do it. Many people will help you learn the skills you need. Believe in yourself, work hard, and you will succeed.

Chapter Four

HEALTH CONCERNS

"I have to live with what I decide."

—*M.P.N.*

Facing Medical Difficulties

When either you or your baby faces a medical difficulty, you feel confused, distraught, and frightened. Worried or angry, you may misunderstand information, jump to conclusions, or confuse old wives' tales with facts. You need to be clear about everything your doctor is saying and to stay well informed.

Doctors handle medical difficulties in different ways. Your doctor may give you general information or make sweeping statements in an attempt to simplify information so you understand it. A pessimistic doctor will exaggerate the incidence or severity of problems and may make things sound worse than they are.

Protective doctors tell their patients very little. This lack of information will leave you feeling stupid and confused. A doctor may expect you to go along with a decision without questioning it.

ASK QUESTIONS

Help your doctor to treat you with intelligence and respect. Ask questions! You have a right to information. Appendix E lists several questions to ask. If questioning your doctor makes you uneasy, have a confidant, partner, or PREGNANCY AIDgency volunteer ask questions for you.

Make sure that you receive complete information about the medical problem, and expect specific answers to your questions. Ask to see literature on the problem, and read it. If you don't understand it, ask a nurse, your doctor, or another doctor to explain it. If the material is even slightly outdated (three to five years old), request current information.

Your treatment should reflect the latest research. National groups that deal with your problem are familiar with up-to-date material and the latest treatments. These groups may also be able to refer you to hospitals or physicians that specialize in treating your problem. Appendix H lists many of these groups.

> *Georgette was three months pregnant with her fourth child when doctors diagnosed Hodgkin's disease, a cancer of the lymphatic system. Since chemotherapy would probably cause the spontaneous abortion of the baby, three doctors recommended abortion followed by chemotherapy or radiation treatment.*
>
> *Frightened, Georgette and her husband prayed and sought the prayers of others. Eventually, at a large, nationally known cancer treatment center, a specialist suggested that Georgette receive small dosages of a single anti-cancer medication, deliver her baby two months early by Cesarean section, and then receive more aggressive treatment. When Georgette's doctor refused to administer this "radical" treatment, she found another who would. Georgette gave birth to a healthy daughter, then began her treatments. Today mother and baby are doing well.*

RECORD INTERVIEWS WITH HEALTH CARE PROFESSIONALS

Take along a tape recorder and ask your doctor's permission to record the advice you hear. Or ask the physician to write down, legibly, *all* instructions, statistics, reference material, predictions, and any other information. Or have the doctor speak slowly and write it down yourself. Read what you have written back to your doctor. Ask about unclear or missing information, and make corrections or additions.

Suppose your doctor is uncooperative and says, "I'm too busy," or "You wouldn't understand." Suppose you're dubbed a "difficult patient" or a "bother." Consider switching doctors. You have a right to ask questions, receive answers, and record information.

At home, review your interview with a confidant, partner, or PREGNANCY AIDgency volunteer. Do you understand it? What other questions do you have? Don't be afraid to keep asking questions until all of your concerns have been addressed. You have a right to know the facts and make your own decisions.

SECOND OPINIONS

Always obtain a second and possibly a third medical opinion of how to best treat your problem. Don't ask your doctor for a referral! Your physician may refer you to someone with views similar to his or her own, or may call the doctor and review your case and prognosis before you set foot in the office. Ask a nurse, confidant, PREGNANCY AIDgency, or support group dealing with your problem for a referral to another doctor for a second opinion, or use the phone book to find one. Don't tell your primary doctor that you are seeking a second opinion. Tell your doctor that you'll call back with your decision.

Don't tell one doctor what another doctor told you. Allow each doctor to make an unbiased diagnosis. Ask each doctor the same questions and record the answers. If you've had tests done, ask each doctor to review the test results with you. Tell the other doctors you've consulted that you'll review what they've said and get back to them.

In the privacy of your home, compare the various opinions and discuss them with your partner, confidant, or PREGNANCY AIDgency volunteer. What are the similarities? Are there any radical differences? Are the opinions based on current information? What options does each doctor suggest?

Return to the doctors and ask them about the differences in treatment without naming the other doctors you consulted. One doctor's name may influence another doctor's opinion. Record what each one says. Choose a doctor who seems optimistic, helpful, and knowledgeable, and who will treat you as you wish. Have any necessary records or tests sent to your new doctor.

Edith and Tracy both had doctors who refused to treat them unless they got abortions.

Without knowing that she was pregnant, Edith had undergone radioisotope testing. Her doctor predicted that her baby was "a severely damaged cretin." Edith had suffered extreme guilt, depression, and psychological problems over a previous abortion. She did not want to go through the mental turmoil again.

Mother of one child, Tracy had severe heart problems and two metal valves in her heart. Six doctors predicted that her second pregnancy would kill her. Tracy didn't care. She wanted her baby to have a chance.

Both women found other doctors, with Tracy calling every physician in the phone book before she found one who would treat her heart condition while managing her pregnancy. Both women had healthy babies and are doing well today.

If you can't find a doctor to agree with the treatment you want, have a legal form prepared. This form should state the medical facts as the doctor sees them, a prognosis, and recommendations. A few sentences will clarify that you have read and understood the doctor's statement, but are choosing not to follow the doctor's suggestions. By taking over your own treatment, you free the doctor from malpractice suits should anything go wrong. To be treated, you must sign the form. Even though you do sign, your doctor still must treat you professionally, within the guidelines of good medical practice.

MEDICAL TESTING

Today, many hospital tests are available to the woman and baby facing medical difficulties. Your doctor should schedule these to determine whether a suspected problem exists and to establish its severity, if possible. Never make a decision based only on opinion. Your medical problem may require any number of tests. A later section of this chapter discusses the more common tests performed during pregnancy.

Ask your doctor if there are any risks involved in the tests you will be taking. What are the risks? Can they be minimized? Are there alternate tests?

After you've agreed on a certain diagnostic test, you should first take the test, and then discuss the results with several doctors before deciding on treatment. Don't agree to a certain treatment before you have even taken the test! For example, if you can't have prenatal testing unless you agree to abort a baby having certain problems, either don't have the testing or don't sign any forms stating you'll choose abortion. Always have a test done and discuss the results before deciding on treatment.

Always take the time to *read* a medical consent form before you sign it. Don't take anyone's word for what it says. Question any terms you don't understand before signing.

Testing has its limitations. One limitation of test results is that they may indicate the presence of a problem, but not its severity. For example, tests may indicate that you have toxemia, but cannot predict how your body will handle the disease. A doctor should always hope for the best outcome while treating you to prevent the worst.

Also, tests occasionally give inaccurate results. Perhaps technicians administered the test improperly. Sometimes testing procedures, conditions, or equipment is faulty. A doctor may misread poorly written test results, or a lab may confuse your tests with those of someone else. Other accidents can happen. If test results are unfavorable, request a retest or additional tests.

Nora's amniocentesis indicated that her unborn son had a genetic defect causing severe disability. Her doctor urged her to have an abortion. Nora and her husband were considering all their options, including parenting, foster care, institutional care, and adoption, when a friend suggested a retest. The friend had aborted a perfectly healthy baby on the basis of an erroneous first prenatal test result. Nora's second amniocentesis indicated that the baby was healthy.

MAKING AND ACTING ON YOUR OWN DECISIONS

Despite most medical difficulties, you will probably be able to have your baby. No one can guarantee that your baby will be healthy or that you will not face some difficulties. However, statistics do prove that with proper medical attention, you can almost always give birth without severe damage to your body.

Calling her an "idiot," Rae's doctor refused to treat her when she would not abort her six-week pregnancy and begin chemotherapy for a cancerous lump under her arm. Rae's husband agreed with her doctor's assessment. Rae had to search for another doctor.

Although surgery found the cancer far advanced, Rae refused radiation treatment when her research showed that the dosage would be harmful to her baby.

During her fifth month of pregnancy, Rae went into premature labor, which was averted. However, doctors discovered that Rae's baby was probably dying. The child had a bowel obstruction, fluid in her stomach cavity, and Down Syndrome, a genetic condition causing mental retardation.

Rae almost wished her baby had been born dead. She investigated adoption but could not go through with it. Rae felt that God had a plan for this baby in her life. Born ten weeks early, the infant survived crises and operations.

When Rae became pregnant again, her husband feared that this pregnancy would hasten Rae's death and leave him with one or possibly two children with special needs. Rae forgives her husband for leaving her when she would not abort. With her Down Syndrome daughter doing well in school and her second daughter healthy, Rae is writing a journal for her children so that they will re-member her should her cancer, now in remission, recur and claim her life.

You probably have questions that cannot be answered by test results or your doctor. National organizations specializing in your health problem can provide an-swers. Appendix H lists many organizations. Your area may have support groups or chapters of these organizations. Your doctor may know people who faced problems similar to the ones you are encountering. Ask for their names and phone numbers and speak to a few people who have faced your problem. Ask them for suggestions on how to cope and where to find help. The information you receive will encour-age you, and you'll be amazed at how you can manage your life despite a health problem.

TRIUMPH FROM TRAGEDY

Your pregnancy may not be the normal, healthy, problem-free pregnancy that you had envisioned, but it can still be a new beginning for you and your baby. Be open to possibilities. You may grow stronger by dealing with this medical problem, and may learn some things that can help others in similar situations. You may educate your doctor or others by the way you handle your difficulty. Certainly you did not want this problem, and no one will ever be able to say that it was a good turn of events. But, with courage and faith, you may be able to turn some part of this trag-edy into a small measure of triumph.

> *"Of all the passions, fear weakens judgement most."*
>
> —*Cardinal de Retz,* Memoirs

Confronting Fears About Your Health

If you're afraid to have your baby because of health problems, get the latest infor-mation from your doctor and know your options. Medication, exercise, surgery, relaxation techniques, or vitamin treatments can manage even severe health prob-lems, such as diabetes, most cancers, hepatitis, and multiple sclerosis. You may have to adjust to your disease, but you and your baby should do well.

CONCERNS ABOUT YOUR AGE

You're never too young to have a baby safely. If you can get pregnant, you can safely give birth. Eat nutritiously and your body will mature with the pregnancy and stay healthy. In some cultures, girls as young as twelve marry and have chil-dren.

Most modern doctors agree that you're never too old to have a baby safely, ei-ther. If you're in good physical condition, stay that way. If you're flabby, ask your doctor for tone-up exercises. Eat nutritiously. Modern health care workers and modern medicine can successfully manage pregnancy in older women.

Olga, Mae, and Vicky all became pregnant unexpectedly, gave birth successfully, and are delighted with their children.

A grandmother, forty-four-year-old Olga felt ill on a camping trip, only to later discover that she was pregnant with twins. A career woman married at thirty-five, Mae felt too old to parent but, at forty-five, discovered that her "menopause" was really pregnancy. At forty-eight, Vicky had long ago completed her family when she found that she was pregnant again. She never menstruated again after giving birth.

PREGNANCY PROBLEMS

During your pregnancy, you may experience a problem such as severe nausea, toxemia, or anemia. These conditions are common to many pregnant women. Proper medical care can manage these and other problems. Be firm in your decision to give birth.

Yvette's patient (Chapter Three) and Abby (this chapter) both suffered extreme nausea while pregnant. Even worse was Barb, who underwent two years of artificial insemination with her husband's sperm before she became pregnant. Dehydrated and hospitalized several times because of nausea, Barb missed much work and had relatives care for her house when she had to stay in bed after she almost delivered at five-and-a-half months. Although suffering some problems when born almost a month early, her son is healthy and active today.

Some mothers are just plain miserable while pregnant. Angry and depressed, they want to be left alone to do nothing. Rose felt that way during all her pregnancies, especially her fourth pregnancy, an event that she didn't plan. She was so upset and ill that she couldn't even do housework. With three little boys, the youngest only a year old, she could hardly keep ahead of her work. She hated falling behind while she endured another horrid pregnancy.

If you are like Rose, ask your doctor if vitamins or exercise can help you feel better. Vitamin B injections helped Rose. Ask someone to help with the housework and find someone you can talk to about your problems. Get out of the house. Try to keep a sense of humor, as did Rose and her husband, who did Rose's housework for her. If you struggle along, you, like Rose, will soon have a baby to delight you.

FEAR OF PREGNANCY AND CHILDBIRTH

Horror stories about pregnancy and childbirth can make you afraid to give birth. Maybe you've had a dreadful pregnancy or birth experience and you're afraid now. Fear is a "disease" that increases your chances of nausea, tension, cramping, and unrest. Going into childbirth with fear almost guarantees that the birth will be agony. Fear will tense muscles, fight the birth process, and increase your pain.

Unlike humans, animals experiencing a normal birth rarely cry out. They don't spend their pregnancies worrying about birth, or worry about when they will experience their next contraction during labor. Animals rest between contractions or pace about. By accepting cramping rather than fighting it, birthing animals often experience little pain. Calmness decreases pain.

Even if you want to be "knocked out" during labor, learn to be calm during the entire birth process by attending natural childbirth classes or by reading about natural childbirth. By learning how childbirth works, you will recognize what's normal, and this knowledge will help control your fear. You'll also learn breathing techniques and exercises similar to the relaxation technique in Chapter Two. These help you relax during labor and make the birth process more comfortable. Practice the exercises every day for weeks so that you can do them automatically during labor.

Look for a capable doctor who knows the latest medical and technological advances and who is committed to giving you a good birth experience without overmonitoring and overmanaging your birth. This individual should be able to recognize and act on a problem, but should let you labor naturally otherwise. Ask how your doctor will handle any predictable problems. Then obtain a second opinion. Another doctor may see your case differently.

Your doctor, nurses, fellow mothers, books, and the questions in Appendix E will help you develop a plan for your labor. You needn't repeat any previous horrible birth experiences. Modern medications, drugs, and techniques assure a relatively painless childbirth.

POSTPARTUM DEPRESSION

How will you feel once your baby is born? Half of all women experience some "baby blues" either immediately after giving birth or a few weeks or months later. Usually the sadness, depression, and feelings of being overwhelmed go away in a week or two.

However, you may experience severe, longer-lasting depression. Find a doctor who will understand your emotional pain. You may need medical treatment or counseling. Build a support system of family, friends, or volunteers from a PREGNANCY AIDgency or women's center. Get advice from other women who have had postpartum depression. Some may even help you with your mothering, housekeeping, and other work.

Several family crises, including domestic violence, relocation, grieving, and illness, contributed to Mary Lou's three experiences with postpartum depression. After one birth, she even tried to commit suicide and take her children with her. Hospitalization, counseling, and learning to recognize and meet her own needs after birth have helped Mary Lou become a counselor to other women going through the "baby blues."

HAVING A BABY WITHOUT HAVING A NERVOUS BREAKDOWN

You may be facing stress, pressure, and crises. If so, your pregnancy will add another crisis, and make you feel as if you might have a nervous breakdown. But don't face your crises alone. A PREGNANCY AIDgency can help you and can refer you to additional help.

You should also try tension-reducing exercises, positive thinking skills, and modifying your diet to reduce stress. Use a journal to determine which problems must be met now and which can be dealt with later. Ask the advice of others who have faced similar problems. Try to envision your life a month from now; two months from now; a year from now; two years from now. Just what help do you need? Where can you get it?

Community agencies can help with housing, counseling, employment, financial management, and many other problems, including overcoming addictions. Volunteers from a religious group or PREGNANCY AIDgency can often provide babysitting, housekeeping, transportation, or care for an ill or elderly person who may be depending on you. Adoption agencies and mothers with children can share parenting advice. Let others help you to meet your needs. You'll feel better.

Frieda and Annie both needed encouragement.

Frieda's youngest child was nine and her oldest was pregnant with Frieda's first grandchild when Frieda became pregnant at forty-two. Usually calm-natured, she needed her pregnant daughter to console and encourage her and assure her that she shouldn't worry about neighborhood gossips discussing grandma's having a baby.

A former career woman, Annie felt incompetent, unfulfilled, and exhausted caring for her premature, high-need, fussy twins. With her twins a year-and-a-half old, she hated her current pregnancy, worried how she'd manage, and was so angry with God that she could no longer pray. A PREGNANCY AIDgency sent her to a mental health counselor and a member of the clergy. Annie felt somewhat better, although it wasn't until she went into labor that she felt the need to pray for a vaginal delivery, since she had had to undergo a C-section with twins. After successfully delivering her baby vaginally, Annie immediately fell in love with her newborn.

Both Frieda and Annie deeply love their children and regret the months they spent in worry and depression.

PSYCHOLOGICAL COUNSELING

If you are receiving mental health counseling, you can almost always continue your pregnancy while under treatment, even if your mental health professional disagrees. If you receive help with your pregnancy, which includes making good plans for your baby, abortion is almost never necessary and many times can be psychologically harmful. This is the conclusion of several psychiatrists in Germaine Grisez's book *Abortion: The Myths, the Realities, and the Arguments.* In fact, one of the psychiatrists notes that completing pregnancy often helps in recovery from mental illness.

Whether or not you parent your baby depends on the severity of your illness, your progress toward healing, and your desire. You may need much help in deciding what to do. If parenting is unwise, you can make a good adoption plan. Have a

PREGNANCY AIDgency volunteer visit your mental health professional. The three of you can work out a good plan to deal with your crises. Even though Ivy's psychiatrist and family urged her to abort, she sought pregnancy counseling and shelter, parented her son, and continued her job. Today she is a married career woman studying for an advanced college degree.

If you're facing medical difficulties, your doctor may have a psychologist confirm that you should end your pregnancy. You'll be told that any sane, rational woman would certainly abort. Nonsense! You can be emotionally secure and want to have your baby! With proper pregnancy management you will probably be able to continue your pregnancy. Surround yourself with positive-thinking people. Get other medical opinions, and contact a PREGNANCY AIDgency for help.

> *Marie had severe toxemia during her two pregnancies. Both babies were premature, and one had lasting physical problems. Despite her responsible use of birth control, Marie became pregnant before a scheduled sterilization procedure.*
>
> *Both her doctor and a psychiatrist he consulted told Marie to abort. Her doctor reasoned that she'd probably miscarry anyway, or that her medication would cause her baby to be grossly deformed and retarded. If her baby survived, could Marie and her husband afford to parent a child with multiple disabilities? Marie might die. Who would care for her children? Suppose she had to go to the hospital months before delivery, as she had to do with her other two babies. Could she find a live-in sitter? Marie was still breastfeeding. How could her body support an unborn baby?*
>
> *Marie felt that she would not be pregnant if God had not planned it. When her professional caregivers realized that Marie would not abort, they became supportive.*
>
> *Marie contacted prayer groups, family members, breastfeeding mothers, and friends for prayers and support. She learned that she could continue to breastfeed as long as she ate well and rested. Her husband received a job promotion, higher wages, and better hours. The family purchased a parcel of land on which to build their own home. After three brief hospital stays during the summer, when Marie's mother, a teacher off for the summer, could babysit her two grandchildren, Marie gave birth by routine Cesarean section during her thirty-sixth week of pregnancy. At that time a sterilization procedure was also done.*
>
> *Diagnosed as deaf, blind, and retarded, the infant began to improve at about nine months of age. By the time he was two years old, he was perfectly healthy. Doctors wonder if Marie's medication had "drugged" her son and kept him from responding until the medication very slowly worked out of his system. Despite some lingering kidney problems, Marie is doing well, and enjoying her children and her new home.*

WHEN YOU HAVE A DISABILITY

Do you have what society calls a "disability"? If so, you know that you're more "differently abled" than "disabled." You've learned to manage your problems with medication, technology, or sheer determination. Many women with a variety of physical limitations have given birth. Many are parenting. Some have spouses who also have physical limitations, yet both manage to be excellent parents, often to perfectly normal children. The human spirit is far more creative than people generally believe. You can bear your baby if you have, as a pastor with a disability said, "the want to."

Your greatest problem may be convincing others that you can give birth and decide about parenting. Find a positive-thinking doctor. Contact a PREGNANCY AIDgency for help. If you are considering adoption, contact an adoption agency. If you want to parent, speak to your doctor or to counseling agencies that treat or raise money for people with disabilities. Ask these individuals for the names of other parents with disabilities. Talking to these parents will inspire you. Your support network will help convince negative thinkers that you can make good plans for your baby.

Stephanie bore and raised three children while suffering from severe, chronic arthritis. Ursa, a victim of multiple sclerosis, had her third child without her disease progressing more rapidly, despite what her doctors predicted. Jenny, who had artificial arms and legs, bore and raised a child conceived as a result of rape. Stephanie received support from her mother and sister; Ursa, from her husband; and Jenny, from a PREGNANCY AIDgency.

Health is a gift we can give ourselves, especially in pregnancy. Even though you may have health problems no matter what you do, you can ease some or all of the problems if you know how. Discuss your health concerns with a doctor, and possibly other professionals, such as mental health workers and nurses. With proper exercise, a good diet, prenatal vitamins, appropriate medications, counseling, and childbirth instruction, you should be able to give birth without permanent harm to either your physical or mental state.

"We fear what we do not understand."

—M.P.N.

Confronting Fears About Your Baby's Health

Every woman wants to have the perfect child, but do you know anyone who has a perfect child? Even the most beautiful child may be stubborn. An intelligent youngster may be shy. A super athlete may have a "swollen head." A generous, kind child may be forgetful or careless.

Every person has some kind of disability. No one succeeds at everything. You build your life around what you *can* do, not around what you *can't*. All children must learn to live with their disabilities, to accept themselves, and to build on their own unique strengths. All parents should love and appreciate their children for who they are. Your children can reach only their own potential, not someone else's.

You may be worried that your unborn child has a *special need*, that is, a physical or mental disability. Or you may wonder if your child has inherited or contracted a *terminal illness*, that is, an illness that will eventually cause your child's death. Don't take your doctor's word that your child has such a condition. Request prenatal testing. If your child has a special need or a terminal illness, refer to Chapter Seven to learn about various parenting plans for children with these problems.

Children with special needs or terminal illnesses require special love. They are neither abnormal nor disabled but limited in activity or cognitive ability, or perhaps both. As one woman with cerebral palsy said, with a smile, "I'm normal for me." Even the child who can neither think nor move responds to love. That's why Dave and Neala have adopted three children with special needs.

WORRIES ABOUT INJURY TO YOUR BABY

If you experience an accident, fall, beating, or other injury, could your baby be harmed? Possibly, but probably not. Your baby is well cushioned in a fluid-filled sac in your womb, so the infant probably felt only a strong jolt. However, if you experience pain in your abdomen or bleeding or discharge from the vagina, or if your child is inactive, speak to your doctor immediately. If you are abused, consider leaving. Refer to Chapter Three.

Will a frightening or stressful experience harm your baby? Probably not, although some believe that prolonged and extreme stress *may* cause long-term physical and emotional problems. But, if you follow the suggestions in this book on managing stress, you should be able to minimize or eliminate its effects. On the other hand, short-term stress should have no effect on your baby's health. Refer to Chapter Two to learn how to release tension and stress.

DRUGS AND MEDICATIONS

Your doctor may be alarmed if you or your partner took any drugs or medications, legal or illegal, before or during pregnancy. Don't let the doctor scare you. Not every drug has an effect on an unborn baby. Those that do don't affect every unborn child exposed to them. The risk depends on the drug, when you took it, how great the dosage, and how often you used it. Your baby probably has a good chance of being healthy. Any problem may be minor, correctable, or reversible.

While taking extremely potent drugs to combat leukemia, Rosemary became pregnant unintentionally. Although her doctor's textbooks indicated that the drugs would almost certainly damage the baby, the child was normal.

Tell your doctor what prescription and over-the-counter medications, drugs, vitamins, salves, powders, and pills you use daily or occasionally. Most are safe. Some may not be. Read labels on drugs and medications to see if they are safe to be taken during pregnancy. If they are not, your doctor can prescribe safe alternatives.

If you take illegal drugs throughout your pregnancy, your baby may be born with a drug addiction and may experience withdrawal. Illegal drugs may cause prematurity, temporary or permanent damage, or death.

If you are using illegal drugs, tell your doctor. You need not worry about being handed over to the police. Instead, your doctor may give you a safer, legal drug, suggest ways for you to cut down your usage, or help you quit using the addictive substance. Drug abuse self-help groups and drug treatment centers can help. End-ing usage now will protect your baby from damage or further damage. With medi-cal help and counseling, Winnie gave up prostitution and a drug habit when she became pregnant. The drug's side effects on her son, who was adopted, were tem-porary.

If your partner is taking drugs, but you are not, then your baby is probably fine. Your doctor can answer your questions. However, seriously consider whether you want a drug addict to parent your child. Although Elaine's husband had a severe drug habit, her baby was not only healthy, but gifted in intelligence. Elaine filed for divorce, moved in with her parents, and continued her education and career while parenting.

ENVIRONMENTAL INFLUENCES

If you were exposed to harmful chemicals, toxic waste, or X rays, your baby may have been damaged, but probably was not. Risk is small even if the exposure was great. Minimize any future risk by avoiding these dangers.

If you're exposed to chemicals or radiation at work, your doctor may suggest ways to minimize your exposure. Although the government may designate the level of exposure as safe, your doctor may feel otherwise. If so, show your employer your doctor's information. Ask a PREGNANCY AIDgency to act as advocate for you. Request a different job within the same company for the remainder of your pregnancy, or ask for additional protection from the harmful substances. You may want to request a leave of absence. Most employers will comply with a doctor's suggestions. They don't want a lawsuit should your baby be harmed.

If you have been exposed to X rays or radioisotopes in a medical setting, your child is probably normal. Any damage could be very slight. Edith, whose story ap-pears earlier in this chapter, underwent radioisotope treatment when pregnant. Her child was normal. Unaware that she was pregnant, Patty had X rays to check a back injury. Despite her doctor's gloomy predictions, her baby was unharmed.

CONCERNS ABOUT USING VIDEO DISPLAY TERMINALS (VDT'S)

Some evidence indicates that working at a video display terminal (computer screen) for a *long* time and under *certain* conditions *might* increase your chance of having a miscarriage or a child with birth defects. Some researchers feel that poor seating posture can impede blood flow to the placenta. Others wonder if low radiation lev-els or weak electromagnetic fields emitted by the monitor in particular may affect oxygen transfer to your baby or be harmful to your baby's development. The more time you spend at the VDT, the greater the problem. If others are using VDT's nearby, you are exposed to radiation and electromagnetism from their VDT's as well as from your own. Most researchers agree that the effect of radiation or elec-tromagnetism decreases with your distance from VDT's. Dr. John Ott's prelimi-nary work indicates that exposing yourself to natural light seems to cancel out some of the effects of electromagnetic fields. More research is being done.

For now, it is wiser to err on the side of safety. The following precautions may set your mind at ease. Discuss them with your employer and doctor.

- Switch to another job that does not use VDT's. Or limit your time at the VDT to less than twenty hours a week—that's four hours a day, five days a week.
- Sit as far away from the monitor screen as possible, using a small table to hold the keyboard. Fit a combination glare and radiation shielding screen over the monitor. Or use equipment for the vision-impaired that enlarges the images on the monitor screen and allows you to sit even farther away.
- Work as far away from other monitors and as close to a natural light source as you can. For example, sit by a window with the drapes open.
- Have fluorescent lights in the work place replaced with full-spectrum, radiation-shielded fluorescent lighting.
- Try to switch to new computer models, put out by some firms, which have the highest radiation shielding.
- Researcher John Ott has observed that monitor-generated electromagnetic fields seem to magnetize the hemoglobin of red blood cells, causing them to clump together abnormally. This probably affects the transfer of oxygen in your body, including the supply to your baby. To minimize this effect, ask your doctor for a prenatal vitamin that has the lowest amount of iron beneficial for pregnancy, and follow the other suggestions listed here.
- Maintain good posture while sitting at the VDT. After using the VDT for forty-five minutes to an hour, get up, stretch, and walk around.
- Daily, spend time outdoors in natural light. You might take your lunch break outdoors.
- Watch the media to keep abreast of the latest developments concerning VDT use during pregnancy.

DISEASES

Your exposure to most diseases will not harm your baby. Check with your doctor to be sure that any medications you're taking are safe.

Exposure to rubella (German measles) early in pregnancy *may* cause birth defects, some major. However, 50 percent of babies exposed to rubella are perfectly normal. Bernice (Chapter Three) and Virginia and Isabel (this chapter) were exposed to rubella early in pregnancy and had normal babies.

Lyme disease, which is carried by infected deer ticks, will harm you and your baby if untreated. If you have Lyme disease, antibiotic treatment will protect you both.

One disease that people can contract without realizing they have it is toxoplasmosis, a disease caused by a parasite whose infectious cysts can be found in the feces of infected cats and possibly in their fur. You can also get toxoplasmosis by eating undercooked fish or meat. Don't feed your cat raw meat. Let someone else clean the cat's litter box. You may not even want to play with your cat, especially if it roams outdoors. Eat only well-cooked meat and fish. Toxoplasmosis affects only

1 in 8,000 babies yearly, and doctors can successfully treat it in most babies before it has devastating effects.

AIDS

AIDS is an incurable disease that eventually causes death. You can get AIDS from sharing drug needles with, receiving a blood transfusion from, or having intercourse with someone who has AIDS. An AIDS-infected mother can give her baby AIDS. If you do not have AIDS but your baby's father does, your baby will be safe. However, ask a doctor or a health clinic about ways to protect yourself from AIDS.

If you do have AIDS, your baby's bloodstream may contain AIDS antibodies. If these antibodies are present, your infant may or may not actually develop AIDS. Blood tests can determine if your baby has the antibodies, but cannot determine if your baby will develop AIDS. Children who do develop AIDS often die young. However, certain effective treatments are helping children live longer.

If you have AIDS, you may prefer to make an adoption or alternate parenting plan. A loving family or group home will parent your child while you may be too weak to do so.

You can parent your child if you have AIDS, although you should not breastfeed. AIDS may be passed from mothers with the virus to babies during breastfeeding. Speak to a health care professional about parenting precautions. By being careful, you can protect your child. Perhaps a doctor or hospital can refer you to an AIDS support group. Here you can talk with others who have AIDS, as well as those working with AIDS victims. You will receive support, advice, and help.

As you get too ill to parent, you may arrange for relatives or friends to care for your child. Or, you may consider adoption, foster care, or one of the group homes that exist for children and their mothers who have AIDS.

> *Caroline, Trini, and Betty all have AIDS, contracted from intravenous drug use.*
>
> *Caroline released for adoption her drug-addicted baby, who had AIDS antibodies in her blood. Adopted by her foster mother, the baby tested negative for the AIDS virus at fourteen months of age.*
>
> *Trini is now drug free and parenting her two children, neither of whom has AIDS. Extremely careful, she scrubs her house with bleach and wears rubber gloves to prevent transmission of the virus. She belongs to an AIDS support group and knows that her family will care for her children when she can't.*
>
> *Weakening from the disease, Betty is only in her twenties. Her boyfriend plans to parent his son, who does not have AIDS.*

Venereal Disease

If you have a venereal disease, your baby is probably all right. You should, however, see your doctor at once. Untreated venereal disease can be damaging. One in four Americans will contract a sexually transmitted disease (STD). If you are sexually active, have your doctor test you for a venereal disease. Call your doctor's attention to any unusual pains or lumps in the abdomen, vaginal discharges, pain upon urination, nausea, fever, or aches. Let your doctor examine any growths, sores, or ulcers in the genital area or elsewhere on your body. Any one of these may indicate a sexually transmitted disease.

Many STDs can be treated successfully without harm to your baby. If you are already under treatment, ask your doctor if your medications are safe to use during pregnancy. You may have to take certain precautions, either before or after birth, depending on the disease. If the disease could have harmed your child, refer to Chapter Seven. However, early treatment generally prevents harm to a baby.

SMOKING

The U.S. Surgeon General warns: "Smoking By Pregnant Women May Result in Fetal Injury, Premature Birth, And Low Birth Weight." The more you smoke, the greater the risk. Breast-fed babies of smoking mothers have a greater chance of being colicky, crying babies. Children who live with parents who smoke have more respiratory illnesses than children of nonsmokers. One survey found that women who smoked during pregnancy were twice as likely as nonsmokers to lose infants after birth to sudden infant death syndrome.

Smoking decreases vitamin C and vitamin B-12 in your blood. If you continue to smoke, ask your doctor about taking supplements of these vitamins. If you smoke to calm yourself down, stay away from chocolate, soft drinks, tea, and coffee. The caffeine in these products may make you nervous and cause you to smoke more.

Pregnancy is the perfect time to stop smoking or to cut back. The earlier you do it, the better for your baby. Your doctor or hospital may be able to refer you to stop-smoking programs. If you are considering a program that involves the taking of antismoking pills or medications, ask your doctor if they are safe for the baby. We all know women who smoked heavily during pregnancy and had healthy babies. However, it's always safer to stop, as Isabel did during her two pregnancies. Both her children were gifted. Unfortunately, Isabel lived with an unpredictable, financially insecure alcoholic husband. After each pregnancy, she began smoking again to "calm herself down," and she died of lung cancer in her mid-forties.

ALCOHOL

Alcoholic beverages are high in calories, and drinking them puts on unnecessary weight. Even worse, alcohol is bad for your baby. The United States Government and several health-related organizations ask all pregnant women to abstain from alcohol. Out of every 100 women who drink heavily throughout their pregnancies, 2 babies will suffer from fetal alcohol syndrome, which causes poor motor development and mental retardation. Out of 100 women who drink any amount of alcohol at all during pregnancy, 3 babies will have problems ranging from low birth weight to spontaneous abortion (death) of the baby.

Even though 95 women out of 100 who drink alcohol at all will have healthy children, pregnancy is still an excellent time to stop drinking. If you can't stop, at least cut back or water down your drinks. Speak to your doctor, hospital, or alcohol abusers support group for suggestions on "drying out." Why put your baby at risk?

Unmarried, alcoholic Vanessa used a PREGNANCY AIDgency to refer her to medical care and shelter as she drank her way through two pregnancies. Years after making adoption plans for her two perfectly healthy children, Vanessa joined Alcoholics Anonymous and sobered up. Still sober, she now supervises a large apartment building and visits one of her children, whom her parents adopted.

WEIGHT PROBLEMS

If you've been dieting, could diet pills, medications, or rapid weight loss have harmed your baby? Speak to your doctor. Your baby is probably fine.

Eating disorders will also affect your health and the health of your baby. Anorexia (eating so little that you become dangerously thin) and bulimia (gorging and then purging with laxatives and vomiting) are addictions that require professional help to overcome. You can combat these problems while pregnant, but you will need professional help. Your doctor can refer you to a good counselor or professional treatment program.

Overweight women usually give birth to perfectly normal babies, but their pregnancies may need some special management. Your doctor can advise you.

If you have weight concerns, ask your doctor for a nutritious diet and an exercise plan. The weight you gain will come off easily after birth. A diet center or supervised diet program can also provide you with diet plans for pregnancy. Exercise programs for pregnant women at the local gym or prenatal clinic can also help prevent weight gain.

BIRTH CONTROL METHODS

When birth control fails and a woman gets pregnant, she often gets just plain mad. Pregnancy was *not* supposed to happen.

Ask your doctor about the failure rate of your method of birth control. Were you using the method correctly? Should you switch methods? What chances do you have of getting pregnant, unexpectedly, again? Most birth control methods, used correctly and consistently, work well. This accidental pregnancy is probably a once-in-a-lifetime event. You will be making once-in-a-lifetime decisions.

Did the birth control method, device, or medication that you were using when you became pregnant harm your baby? Probably not. If you have fears about your baby's health, speak to your doctor. The questions in Appendix E may help. Ask to see professional literature and statistics. You may consider prenatal testing. Refer to Chapter Seven on parenting plans for a child with special needs or a terminal illness.

If you conceived with an IUD (intrauterine device) in place, tell your doctor. The doctor will make sure that your baby is not growing outside the uterus—a dangerous situation. The doctor will probably be able to remove the IUD without harming the baby. If not, you can continue the pregnancy with the IUD in place, although you will have an increased chance of miscarriage. The presence of an IUD should not cause deformities in your baby.

With two sons in school, Iris was planning to get a graduate degree and return to teaching to help pay off their two-bedroom house and several bills. Despite using an IUD, she noticed with dismay the familiar signs of pregnancy. When her doctor wanted to do a D & C, a procedure to empty her womb, Iris insisted on a pregnancy test first. Doctors were unable to remove the IUD without disturbing the pregnancy, so Iris had to rest to control spotty bleeding. She worried about her baby's having a disability and about her family's small house and tight budget. Her son is a healthy child who delights his family.

Using a condom or diaphragm will not harm your baby. With these birth control methods, you may also use a spermicide cream, jelly, or suppository. There are some who say that spermicides may cause birth defects, but studies are not in agreement about this. If spermicides caused a vast, obvious increase in birth defects, many studies should have shown it. The chance of spermicides' harming your baby is probably small.

If you conceived while using oral contraceptives, prenatal testing can determine what damage, if any, has actually occurred. Stop taking birth control pills and see your doctor if you think you are pregnant. Most babies conceived while their mothers were taking the pill are perfectly normal.

Perhaps you conceived while using natural family planning, as Faith did (Chapter Three), or after a vasectomy, as happened to Vera (Chapter Three). These should not have harmed your baby.

AGE CONCERNS

Being very young doesn't put you at any extra risk of having a child with special needs or medical difficulties as long as you eat well and take care of your health. Your baby should be fine. Fourteen-year-old Lucy ate well throughout her pregnancy, ignored her boyfriend's pressure to abort, and had a healthy, normal son whom she is raising in her parents' home.

The older you get, the slightly greater chance you have of bearing a child with Down Syndrome. If you are forty, you have a 2 percent chance of bearing a child with Down Syndrome. If you are forty-five, you have a 3 percent chance; if forty-nine, a 9 percent chance. This means that of every 100 women who get pregnant at age forty-nine, 91 will have babies *without* Down Syndrome.

Children born with Down Syndrome are mildly or moderately mentally retarded, and have characteristic facial features. Some have additional health problems, but Down children born today have a life expectancy of fifty-five years. With infant stimulation and proper education, Down Syndrome children can learn to read and write and can become self-supporting, happy citizens. A letter written by an adult with Down Syndrome appears in Appendix B.

A child with Down Syndrome has an excellent chance of a good and satisfying life. If you cannot raise your child, many couples are waiting to adopt Down Syndrome children.

If you're an older mother, your chance of having a child with a genetic condition other than Down Syndrome is probably no greater than a younger woman's chances. Mae, Olga, and Vicky (earlier in this chapter) are older mothers who had perfectly normal children.

RH FACTOR

If your blood type is Rh negative, your baby may be in danger of blood disease, brain damage, and possibly death if left untreated. Tell your doctor about any previous pregnancies, whether they ended in birth, miscarriage, or abortion, and about any blood transfusions. Doctors can successfully treat your baby. A doctor can also give you a vaccine to prevent Rh disease from affecting future children.

INHERITED OR CONGENITAL CONDITIONS

A child may have any number of special needs or health problems. These may be inherited from the parents, or may occur during development in the womb. These conditions can range from mild to severe, and can involve mental or physical growth or both. Be sure that your child's prognosis is as up-to-date as possible.

Misinformation abounds on various diseases. For example, there are those who think that children with hemophilia often bleed to death from minor wounds. The truth is, internal injuries pose a greater risk.

Information can be outdated as well. For years, geneticists believed that any male child conceived with a fragile X chromosome was mentally retarded (females with fragile X are normal or have very minor learning problems). Latest findings show that 10 percent of male children with fragile X are normal. No one knows why.

Doctors may be unaware of the most current treatments. For example, many doctors don't know about the latest, life-prolonging treatments for the serious blood disorders thalassemia and sickle cell anemia. Other doctors still think that spina bifida children are hopelessly incurable, but modern treatments can help most spina bifida infants to mature into independent adults who can hold down jobs.

Ask professionals for the most *current* literature. Refer to other parts of this chapter for additional information. Call national agencies, which have the latest information on your child's problems. Some agencies are listed in Appendix H. Be sure that the prognosis you hear considers current medical treatments.

Doctors told Gala and Odessa that their spina bifida babies were severely damaged and dying, and recommended nontreatment. Instead, Odessa contacted a modern children's hospital that treated the baby. Today Odessa's child walks and has normal intelligence. Gala insisted on treatment for her son at birth and re-

ceived help through a charity for special needs children. Her son, though mentally retarded, can talk clearly and direct his wheelchair.

The information you receive regarding the physical and mental consequences of the condition affecting your child should be complete as well as accurate. For example, Turner's syndrome has no effect on a girl's intelligence but will keep her body from physically maturing unless she receives hormonal treatments.

Surgery can help many conditions. Congenital heart defects, for example, can often be treated through surgery or with drugs, either before or after birth.

A rapidly expanding home health care industry makes many conditions treatable in the home. For example, children with cystic fibrosis can use portable, pocket-sized pumps to administer antibiotics continuously to fight dangerous lung infections. Insurance usually pays for home health care and equipment.

A victim of Carpenters Syndrome, Cecilia's newborn had severe bone deformities. Doctors said that he was mentally retarded, probably severely so, and would likely die. However, when the baby did well with an oxygen unit, doctors reconstructed his skull, allowing room for brain growth. Other operations followed. Today the boy is speech-delayed, not mentally retarded, breathes on his own, and has a near-normal appearance. Cecilia and her husband were grateful for the prayers of family, friends, and church members, and for their financial support and generous gifts.

If you or your partner has a problematic condition that your baby could inherit, people may discourage you from having a child. Should you get pregnant, doctors may urge you to submit to genetic testing. If your child has special needs or certain health problems, you may be pressured to abort. Yet who can better teach your child how to live with the condition than you? If you choose to make an adoption plan for your baby, who can write your child a letter of encouragement better than you?

Charlotte had struggled to find acceptance despite a very visible physical disability. When prenatal tests showed that her daughter had the same physical deformity, Charlotte refused her doctor's suggestions of abortion. She and her husband plan to teach their daughter that what people do with their lives is more important than appearance.

Any condition in the parents that occurred because of accident, environmental influence, or disease is not hereditary.

Most emotional disorders are not inherited. Even with those that could be, only a small percentage of children will develop the illness. Even if both parents have schizophrenia, their child still has no more than a 50 percent chance of developing the disease. Schizophrenia and other mental disorders can usually be treated successfully with medication, counseling, and sometimes hospitalization for periods of time.

Certain physical conditions and tendencies toward chronic illness and IQ levels may be inherited, but not as often as commonly thought. As discussed in Appendix C, many mentally retarded women can conceive normal babies and can give birth. With early childhood stimulation and education, children can increase their IQ. Proper diet and other treatments may help control certain chronic conditions. A child who inherits a disability or a health problem may have a milder form than either parent has. Your child will have an excellent chance for treatment, as doctors can diagnose the condition early and begin treatment immediately.

NEW FRONTIERS

Doctors at many large university center hospitals are now performing some types of fetal surgery to correct life-threatening conditions in the unborn child. Despite the risks involved, fetal surgery has saved unborn babies. Four-and-a-half months after conception, unborn baby Amy Spencer was operated on to drain a life-threatening cyst. When she was born seventeen weeks later, the drain was removed. A twenty-three-week-old unborn child, Baby Mitchell was successfully operated on for a blocked urinary tract, then returned to his mother's womb to finish development until birth.

Your baby may need an organ transplant. However, you may have to be aggressive in order to have your child receive this costly operation. Going public with your needs elicits sympathy and help, and may make the transplant possible.

> When their newborn needed a liver transplant, Wallis and her husband mounted an effective, tiring media campaign in which even professional sports players and actors brought public attention to their plight. With strangers sending in funds and the family's insurance company amending its policy to include liver transplants, the parents were able to get their baby a liver. A year and a half later, he is an active, healthy two-year-old.

CHARTING A COURSE OF ACTION

Concern about your baby's health is natural. Learn which fears are groundless and which are a real cause for concern.

If you have fears, talk to your doctor about them. Determine what chance you actually have of bearing a child with special needs. Consider prenatal testing if you are especially concerned. If your child has special needs or health problems, review all your parenting options, as discussed in Chapters Five and Seven. Knowledge about risks, prognoses, parenting options, and up-to-date treatments can help you make decisions without fear.

"Today wombs have windows."

—M.P.N.

Choosing Prenatal Testing

Sometimes doctors suggest ending a pregnancy because a problem *may* exist. Has your doctor told you that your baby will "probably" or "definitely" be "retarded" or "deformed"? How does your doctor know?

Years ago no one knew if a baby had special needs or health problems until birth or even months or years later. Today, prenatal tests check your baby before birth. If something might be wrong with your baby, your doctor should test to be sure. Would a doctor operate for lung cancer just because it *seemed* as if you had it? A good doctor would find out for sure, then operate.

> *When Virginia was one month pregnant, her two-year-old caught rubella (German measles). When Virginia, a nurse, asked for a gamma globulin injection to protect her baby, her obstetrician said, "Your baby's been exposed and is going to be deaf, blind, retarded, or dead anyway. The gamma globulin won't do any good." So Virginia called another doctor who gave her the injection and took a blood test which indicated that the virus could have affected the baby. Virginia's original doctor said, "You don't have to have the baby. I could recommend someone to you."*
>
> *Virginia credits her faith in God for sustaining her through nine months of worry before she gave birth to a perfectly healthy baby.*

You'll probably be asked to take at least one prenatal test. You need to know if you want it.

Prenatal testing can be expensive. Ask your doctor about the cost. Will your insurance cover it? If not, can you afford the test? Can less expensive tests be done? If your insurance does cover the cost of prenatal tests, your doctor may schedule many of them. Do you want to submit to all of these? Are they necessary?

Prenatal testing cannot detect every possible problem or guarantee the "perfect" child. No prenatal test is 100 percent accurate. Some tests carry a greater probability of error than others. Some rely on a doctor to interpret the results. A borderline result may indicate a problem to one doctor and no problem to another doctor. Sometimes testing indicates a problem when none is present. If tests indicate a problem, ask for a retest or additional tests, as did Nora, whose story appears earlier in this chapter.

> *Estelle and Abby had more than one prenatal test.*
>
> *When Estelle's alphafetoprotein (AFP) test results were abnormally low, her family and friends urged her to abort her baby, who her doctor thought would be malformed and probably grossly retarded. However, amniocentesis showed that the baby was normal but two weeks younger than the doctor had thought.*
>
> *During her seventh pregnancy, Abby gained excessive weight too quickly and became so weak and nauseated that she had to be hospitalized twice. Ultrasound revealed twins, one of which was dead and being reabsorbed. Because the other twin could die, and because Abby had a benign uterine tumor that had caused her to miscarry previously, her doctor monitored the pregnancy with several tests. Some professionals felt that the tests indicated spina bifida, external body intestines, and mental retardation in the surviving twin. Abby's doctor said that the baby was fine. Abby's premature labor was averted, and she gave birth to a healthy daughter.*

Have your child tested after birth to confirm the results of prenatal tests. Testing after birth almost always yields accurate results, although in rare cases this testing, too, may be wrong. Doctors told Marie, whose story appears in this chapter, that her baby had permanent problems. Today he is perfectly healthy.

THE LIMITS OF PRENATAL TESTING

The following is a list of what prenatal testing *cannot* do.

- Prenatal testing cannot discover emotional or behavioral problems. A clinically "normal" child may have emotional or behavioral problems, while a child with a disability or illness might be emotionally stable.
- Prenatal testing often cannot indicate the severity of a problem. It may be possible to determine the severity only after birth.
- Prenatal testing cannot predict exact IQ levels. Many mentally retarded children exceed expectations.
- Prenatal testing cannot always accurately predict how long a dying baby will live. You can get an idea but really can't be sure.
- Some prenatal tests indicate that a child *could* have a problem, not that a child *does* have a problem. For example, Duchenne muscular dystrophy is a progressive, fatal disease that affects boys only. When a pregnant woman carries the gene for this disease, prenatal tests can determine if her baby is a boy, but only tests after birth can determine if he has the illness.
- Prenatal testing cannot tell you what to do about a problem. Knowing about a problem can help you explore parenting and treatment options, but you could do this after birth if you didn't have the testing.
- Prenatal testing cannot predict how your child will handle problems. It cannot predict if someone, soon, will find a new treatment or cure for your child's condition. Prenatal testing can't measure the parenting environment or tell which people, perhaps including yourself, can love and help your child.

TREATABLE OR NOT?

If your doctor wants to schedule a test, ask why, then decide if the reason given warrants the test.

Testing may reveal a problem that can be treated before birth. However, most children with special needs or health problems can be treated only after birth, and some problems have no cures or treatments.

Some mothers, like Darlene (Chapter Seven), feel that certain doctors treat an unborn child known to have special needs or certain health problems less aggressively than a "normal" baby who is in danger. Since Darlene feels that unfavorable test results prejudiced her doctor against aggressively treating her unborn baby, she refused prenatal testing in a subsequent pregnancy. If your doctor is testing for an untreatable problem, do you want the test?

If birth problems such as prematurity, postmaturity, or Cesarean section threaten, a doctor may use prenatal tests to determine if a baby could be safely born or if special equipment must be used. This can protect your baby's life.

Some doctors schedule tests to confirm stages of pregnancy and to look for dangerous conditions, as Abby's doctor (earlier in this chapter) did. This can help them better manage your pregnancy.

Prenatal testing carries some minor risks to both mother and baby. Is your desire to know the health of your baby worth the small risk involved with testing?

Laura, Rita, and Trudy all faced prenatal testing.

Laura had an increased risk of having a mentally retarded child since she was forty years old and both she and her husband had mentally retarded relatives. However, she planned to parent her child no matter what, so she refused prenatal testing. Her child is classified as a genius.

Since Rita (Chapter Seven) had a daughter who was born with a fatal genetic condition, she had prenatal testing during the following pregnancy to prepare for the child's birth in case of another problem. However, this baby was normal.

After having three miscarriages, Trudy was half afraid to try again for another child. Although doctors monitored her pregnancy with ultrasound, she refused all other prenatal tests, since she wanted to have her baby and in no way endanger the pregnancy. She gave birth to a healthy girl.

SELECTING A PRENATAL TEST

What tests are you contemplating? Ask your doctor to explain each test and the stage of pregnancy at which it is done. Inquire about the test's risks and benefits, its accuracy and percentage of error, and what it can and cannot reveal. Ask if treatments are available for any problems found. Don't accept general reassurances—get percentages and specific information. Evaluate, then decide what to do.

Ask to speak to other women who have had the test. They will tell you what it *really* was like! Doctors tell patients that amniocentesis doesn't hurt, but it hurt Darlene, whose story appears later. She also had contractions for three days following the test. Doctors say this is a "normal side effect," but it causes a spontaneous abortion of 1 out of every 100 babies. A good doctor will tell you that, too.

Types of Tests

Ultrasound bounces high-frequency sound waves off your baby and reflects your child's image onto a screen. Ultrasound is almost routinely done today and often is an aid to the safe delivery of a baby. While checking on a baby's health, ultrasound also can determine a child's gestational age and position in the uterus and can confirm the presence of twins.

Some scientists wonder if ultrasound waves may cause some undetected damage to the developing child's body cells. However, no evidence of damage has yet been found. Ultrasound is only as good as the person reading the screen and interpreting the results. Some untrained doctors have misread a baby's sex or incorrectly interpreted a problem.

Amniocentesis ("amnio" for short) is done around the sixteenth week of pregnancy. Fetal cells, withdrawn from the womb through a needle, are analyzed for genetic defects. The needle occasionally strikes the baby. This may be partly responsible for the increased risk of pregnancy loss associated with amniocentesis. Amniocentesis also seems to increase the chances of a premature birth and may be associated with an increased susceptibility to inner ear infections in childhood.

In **fetoscopy**, done in mid-pregnancy, an endoscope (large, needle-sized metal tube) illuminates the uterus while a technician takes a sample of your baby's blood or skin for analysis. Fetoscopy seems to increase the rate of spontaneous abortion and premature labor.

Done early in pregnancy, **chorionic villi sampling** uses a catheter inserted into the uterus to obtain a baby's tissue sample for analysis. This tricky procedure increases the chance of miscarriage.

Around the sixteenth to eighteenth week of pregnancy, **alphafetoprotein** (AFP) testing analyzes a mother's blood sample to determine how much AFP, a substance produced by the baby's liver, is present. High or low levels may indicate a genetic problem. Or they may mean that the baby is younger or older than the doctor thought, or that Mom has a problem. If you have unfavorable AFP test results as Estelle (earlier in this chapter) did, get another test to determine if the baby really has a problem. AFP testing is often false-positive on the first try.

In most cases, doctors suggest amniocentesis, fetoscopy, chorionic villi sampling, and AFP tests to determine if an unborn baby is healthy or genetically normal. In many places, these tests are becoming routine. If a baby has special needs or severe health problems, the mother can choose to abort. Many doctors prefer earlier prenatal testing because they feel that aborting earlier in pregnancy is safer physically and less traumatic emotionally for the mother.

Most doctors ask pregnant women to have at least one prenatal test. Since some women have sued doctors for not telling them about prenatal testing, your doctor may pressure you to have a test. However, if a test is not required by law, you can refuse it. You may want to refuse prenatal testing if you would not consider abortion if you don't like the test's risks, or if your doctor is not testing for a problem that could be treated before birth. If your doctor is really pushy, switch doctors, or file a letter with your doctor stating that you refused prenatal testing against doctor's recommendations.

FACING THE BIRTH OF A CHILD WITH
SPECIAL NEEDS OR HEALTH PROBLEMS

Prenatal testing may reveal that your child has special needs, a terminal illness, or abnormalities incompatible with life. Many people, including family members, friends, doctors, nurses, and genetic counselors, believe that women should choose abortion for such children. They may believe that you have a right to a normal child or that you cannot mentally, physically, or financially handle an infant who has certain conditions. Perhaps they feel that people with special needs or terminal illnesses live unhappy lives of lesser quality and are "better off dead." Others feel that caring for people with severe problems requires an unwise use of money and resources.

You may experience tremendous pressure to abort a "less-than-perfect" child. The pressure will probably be greater if the child is dying.

Suddenly everyone's love and concern for your baby becomes rejection. They assume that your love will diminish when you learn that your child has problems. If your child is left with a disability following an accident or is found to be terminally ill after birth, no one expects a parent's love to evaporate. Why should it evaporate for your unborn baby?

Maybe you want to give your baby a chance. A medical team that pressures you to abort will add tremendous stress to your situation. Your very first parenting challenge may be to convince your medical team to let you give birth, or to switch to more supportive doctors. Refer to Chapter Seven for more information on caring for children with health problems or special needs.

DEALING WITH YOUR FEELINGS WHEN YOUR UNBORN BABY HAS A PROBLEM

If you know your baby has special needs or severe health problems, you'll feel strange and helpless as you carry your child within you. You can't run from, heal, see, or touch your baby. Prove your love by talking to your infant now and making plans for the future. Together, you and someone very close to you can tell close relatives and friends about your baby.

But what do you tell casual acquaintances and strangers? Give them information they can handle. Answer their questions briefly and don't embarrass them by mentioning your baby's problem. After answering the question, change the subject.

"I didn't know you were pregnant!"

"I sure am!"

"When's the baby due?"

Give your due date.

"I bet you're glad."

"Yes, I am."

"Do you know if it's a boy or a girl?"

"Don't you like to be surprised? I do." (If you don't mention your baby's sex, you don't have to mention testing results.)

"Did you have prenatal testing?"

"Yes."

"How was it?"

"My baby has a problem but deserves a chance to reach his or her potential. Thanks for your concern."

DO YOU REALLY WANT PRENATAL TESTING?

Now that you know what prenatal testing can and cannot do, you need to answer the question, "Do I want prenatal testing? Why? Why not?"

Only you know what is best for you and your baby. Some women are relieved to know that their children are normal. Others want to make special plans for their children if their children have special needs or health problems. If the baby's problems can't be treated before birth, many women don't want to know about them until the birth. How do you feel? Talk over with your confidant your decision to have or to refuse prenatal testing. Choose the option that will help you to rest easier.

Chapter Five

AFTER THE BIRTH

"We are family, for a lifetime."

—*M.P.N.*

Thinking About Parenting Your Baby

Even if you're married, you don't have to "fall into" parenting. You have a choice. With a partner or confidant, answer the questions in Appendix G. These discuss parenting and adoption options.

If you do parent, expect change. Change can be exciting, joyful, or frustrating, and with a child you will experience all three! What changes will your baby make in your life? Can you adjust? Even if your baby is a surprise, remember that a lot of surprises are happy ones.

> *With her children in school, her family complete, her part-time job fulfilling, and plans underway to enlarge her home, Ellen became pregnant unexpectedly. After overcoming the initial shock, Ellen and her husband Carl got excited about the baby. Ellen worked until her sixth month of pregnancy, then took a break during the business's slow season. At a surprise baby shower, she received many baby items to replace the ones she'd given away. Friends loaned her additional baby furniture and baby clothing.*
>
> *Having breast-fed her other children, Ellen decided to bottle-feed this infant so that she could return to work when her daughter was two months old and Ellen and a friend could exchange babysitting favors. Her baby is now walking, the house addition is completed, and Ellen and her family are very happy.*

If you're divorced or widowed, you're dealing with the crisis of losing your husband. Are you willing and able to parent now? Do you feel a bond with the baby or do you resent the responsibilities of parenting now? Talk over your feelings with someone you can trust, possibly a PREGNANCY AIDgency volunteer, member of the clergy, psychologist, family counselor, or confidant, or another parent. Make plans that are best for you.

> *Polly, mother of one child and on welfare, discovered her pregnancy right after her husband Chad went to live with a girlfriend. She made an appointment for an abortion, then changed her mind as the procedure was beginning. She determined that Chad's behavior would not ruin her life. After giving birth, Polly moved. When Chad found out what had happened, he wanted to return to the marriage. Polly laid down conditions. Chad and Polly would have to move into their own apartment. Chad would have to include Polly in his recreational plans, communicate with Polly, and stop having affairs.*
>
> *Chad met Polly's demands. They are working through hurtful memories for the sake of their children.*

Many single women, like Jo (following), choose to parent their babies. They work hard to resolve the difficulties they face.

> *When Jo was a college freshman, she became pregnant. She didn't want her family to know about her pregnancy. When Jo took her disinterested boyfriend's offer to pay for an abortion, she called a phone number she saw in a newspaper but reached a PREGNANCY AIDgency, not an abortion clinic. The AIDgency volunteer explained the help that would be available if Jo decided to have her baby. Jo took six weeks to decide to give birth.*
>
> *Jo dropped out of college, then found a job. When her job insurance would not pay for pregnancy costs, the AIDgency arranged for free medical care and a lowered hospital fee. Jo probably would have been fired for missing so much work due to nausea, but the AIDgency explained the situation to Jo's employer. Soon Jo felt better and was able to keep working.*
>
> *With the help of the PREGNANCY AIDgency, Jo moved in with a single mother, then into a shelter home, then into a small, affordable apartment furnished with donated furniture. She went for adoption counseling but decided to parent her son. The AIDgency gave Jo maternity clothing, baby clothing, and baby furniture. When Jo returned to work, she placed her son in day care. Eventually, Jo moved back home, where her mother babysat while Jo worked.*

TO MARRY OR NOT?

A parent of seven children advised each of them, "Before you marry, keep both eyes and both ears open. After you marry, close one of each." Sound advice if you're considering marriage because you're pregnant. Choose a mate wisely, then overlook the little faults. If you're considering marriage, refer to Appendix F.

If your baby's father is caring, responsible, and loving, then getting married before your baby is born may work for you. However, many marriages fail when couples tie the knot because the woman is pregnant. It may be better to decide about marriage after the baby is born, when the pressure to marry quickly is gone. If your baby's father would not be a good parent, it might not be wise to marry him just to "give your baby a name" or because you fear no one else will marry you if you have a baby. You may later marry an understanding man.

Debbie, Stacie, and Leona made three different sets of marriage plans.

After living together for several years, Debbie and Bob decided to marry when Debbie became pregnant. They now have two children, share parenting and housekeeping responsibilities, and are very happy.

A recent high school graduate, Stacie visited a PREGNANCY AIDgency and changed her mind about having an abortion. Her boyfriend asked her to postpone an adoption decision. When he got a job and an apartment, Stacie, who had now given birth, married her boyfriend, applied to and was accepted into nursing school, and began her new life as a career mother and wife.

Pregnant in high school, Leona didn't want to marry her baby's immature father, so her mother and father helped her parent while she finished high school and got a job. Later she married a more mature man, who adopted the child.

PARENTING—A LIFETIME OCCUPATION

Parenting a child means being "Mom" for life. Do you know how to parent or how drastically your lifestyle will change if you do? Are you ready for this commitment?

If you've never had any experience with parenting, you may not realize what parenting your child really means. You need to find out what parenting is all about before you can prepare for it. Many high schools provide parenting classes for students; and hospitals and women's centers can refer you to community parenting classes and groups. You should definitely attend one of these groups.

If you don't know how to parent, look for some families who have children and talk to them about what parenting means. Do some babysitting, not just for a few hours but for a day or more at a time. Can you live with the responsibility of parenting a child twenty-four hours a day, year after year? If you are a teen, talk to other teenaged moms who are parenting about how they manage and how they feel about it. If you decide to parent, ask some other parents if you can call them for advice when you have questions or feel frustrated. Then call them, often.

Are you ready to parent a toddler, child, adolescent, teen, young adult? Suppose you decide to parent your child, then realize that you made a mistake. Adoption is *always* an option, no matter what your child's age. Of course, infants adapt better to new families than older children do, but no matter what their age, children are better off with parents who can care for them well. If you recognize that parenting your child was a mistake, admit it, like Olivia did, and do what is best for both you and your child. After struggling with welfare and an unsupportive lover, Olivia asked relatives to adopt her two children. She is working to put her life together and visits her children often.

CHOOSING TO PARENT

Choosing to parent means receiving advice. Learn to sift good advice from bad by reading books and articles on parenting, talking to other parents, and discussing parenting with your partner or confidant.

Ideas on parenting have changed. For example, while child psychologists used to advise women to let babies "cry it out" and to feed them on schedules, today they advise cuddling babies and feeding them on demand. Parents are advised to begin discipline when a child can understand the meaning of the words "no," "not now," and "wait." Toddlers may not *like* these words, but they understand them!

Compare modern and traditional advice, and choose a parenting style that works best for you and your child. You'll make some mistakes—no one is perfect. You may not be able to provide all you would like for your child. However, if you're generous with love, patience, and acceptance, then you're good parent material. Enjoy your child!

"Superwoman never was a mother."

—M.P.N.

Fitting Your Baby Into Your Lifestyle

Babies need a lot of your time, and you can't schedule or postpone their demands. Some mothers, like Cathy, love the job of parenting babies. They really don't mind sleepless nights, dirty diapers, or colicky babies. Mothering is what these women want to do. Although Cathy and her Navy officer husband moved twelve times in three years and had six children in seven years, Cathy felt that parenting was "easy . . . a joy." She felt fulfilled in living totally for her children. Unlike Cathy, you may need time for yourself.

Maybe you do so much for others that you secretly resent it. Wanting time to yourself isn't unloving. You have to satisfy your desires, part of the time, to mother happily.

You may be satisfied to put off certain interests or a career until your children enter nursery school or kindergarten, or you may need time to yourself right now. Be honest. Do you feel that you will go crazy if you have to care for a baby full-time? Do you sometimes feel like a slave to everyone else's needs? Are you afraid of harming one of your children? When exhausted, do you ever feel like running away? Your fear, anger, frustration, and resentment are signs that you need time to do what you like and to discover yourself. You're not Superwoman, so why not admit it?

Ask your partner or friend to babysit for you while you go off alone to assess your needs. Do you need money? Time to yourself? Less housework? Child care? An adult to talk to?

PARENT SUPPORT GROUPS

Other parents often provide the best advice. Talk to some parents to find out how they adjusted to their new situations. Ask a social service organization or church if there are parent support groups available. No matter what your marital status, join both a couple's and single parent's group. Often, group members babysit for each other, exchange children's clothing, car pool, and help each other. Like you, these parents have felt anger, frustration, and despair. They can advise you of how to control strong emotions.

You'll also learn how to keep or resume open communication with a partner. You must take time for each other, time to touch (not just have sex), listen, and share. Pull together and stay together.

Also ask other parents how they introduced a new baby to any jealous household pets or siblings. A veterinarian or animal shelter may also have suggestions on overcoming jealousy in pets. A pediatrician or child psychologist can give you advice on sibling rivalry. Continue to give your pets and other children attention and don't leave the baby alone with them.

CHILD CARE

In order to care for your child, you may need to change the way you are used to living. You may have to rearrange schedules and set priorities. Be daring. As one wise woman said, "If you have trouble meeting your standards, lower your standards." Lynn (Chapter Two) did.

Parents, friends, or relatives can often help with babysitting, a place to live, and child care. Ellen, Jo, and Leona (all earlier in this chapter) asked for help. So did fifteen-year-old Veronica, whose father would not let her come home because she was pregnant. She went to live with her boyfriend's family, married him, and took parenting courses. He finished high school and got a job. The marriage is successful.

If you need a great deal of help, maybe you and a friend can take turns babysitting each other's children. Get your partner to watch the kids. Offer room, board, and a small stipend to a live-in nanny. Hire older children to do chores or to babysit. Maybe you can afford day care, housekeepers, or gardeners.

When Naomi became pregnant in her mid-forties, she learned that her son Alan had Down Syndrome, a genetic condition that causes mental retardation. Naomi said to her husband Marshall, "We can go crazy and get mad at each other, trying to take care of Alan and our other four kids, or we can get help." So they hired a nanny to help Alan do special exercises and to babysit. They lobbied for high-quality special education classes in their school district, and gave Alan swimming and music lessons. Today Alan babysits for his nephews and nieces. One nephew wrote a school essay about Alan entitled "The Person Who Has Most Influenced My Life."

Perhaps you need someone to parent your child for you for a while. Perhaps a relative or friend can do this. Sometimes a religious organization or PREGNANCY AIDgency can find a family to parent for you. Foster care can look after your baby for a few months until you can parent. Persist until you find someone who will help you. You will retain full legal status as the child's mother. The parenting family or foster care family will provide only temporary care.

Two months pregnant and behind in her rent, Anita listened to her landlady's advice and went for an abortion. At the clinic door, she met a pro-life advocate whose religious community offered to pay Anita's back rent, give her money and material help, and care for her baby for months at a time while Anita harvested grapes. After four years of working the grape harvest, Anita decided to return to her parents. A member of the religious community that had been babysitting Anita's child drove Anita and her daughter back to Mexico, where they are now both happily settled.

PARENTING A HOUSEFUL OF YOUNG CHILDREN

A young psychologist and his wife had four children, all preschoolers. When his wife wanted some time to herself, the psychologist volunteered to babysit while his wife went out. After a few hours with four crying, fighting, demanding children, he couldn't wait for his wife to get home. Counseling twenty suicidal patients was a much easier job!

Your children can wear you out. Some of the novel and not-so-novel ideas that follow, successfully used by parents of large families, may help you out.

- Certain baby items and appliances can make life easier when you are caring for children. Thrift shops, secondhand stores, and garage sales often feature these items at inexpensive prices. A PREGNANCY AIDgency can provide free baby items. Be sure that secondhand items meet government safety regulations. Labor-saving baby items include:

  —A baby carrier to carry your baby while you work.
  —A stroller to stroll your baby indoors, with your foot, while you work. You could also let older, responsible children stroll the baby.
  —A baby walker, playpen, and wind-up baby swing.
  —An infant car seat to keep your baby safe while riding in a car and to double as an infant seat in your home. If your baby is overtired or fussy, you can secure the car seat inside your automobile, strap your infant into the car seat, and take a ride. Your baby should fall blissfully asleep.
  —Household appliances (if you can afford them) such as a dishwasher, clothes washer, microwave oven, food processor, and clothes dryer.

- Changes in household routine can make life easier. Try these tips to save work:

  —Teach children to keep toys in one room only.
  —Tidy up the rooms visitors see. Close doors to other rooms. If the house is untidy and the doorbell rings, put the vacuum in the middle of the floor and say you were just cleaning up.
  —Use a diaper service if you can afford it.
  —Clean on schedule, maybe every two weeks.
  —Have someone babysit while you organize your house.
  —Simplify meals.
  —If your kids aren't really dirty, bathe them every other day instead of every day.
  —Use clothes that don't require ironing.

—Launder only dirty clothes. If something looks and smells clean, don't wash it.

—Change sheets and pillowcases less often.

—Play with or read to kids in groups.

—Teach your children personal care skills as soon as they can handle them. Have children help with household tasks and reward them for good work and effort.

—Take time to do something you really like. Keep one social activity. Make time to be alone, too.

—Keep communication open with your partner. Daily or weekly, spend some time together, alone.

—When you put your children down for naps, lie down, too. If they won't sleep, lock them in the room with you with a few toys. Then, lie down and keep an eye on them while you relax.

In two years, your baby will be much more independent. Your other children will be two years older and more responsible. After two years of adjustment, you'll have more time to enjoy your family.

With two sets of twins and two other children, Holly was pregnant with her seventh child when her oldest entered kindergarten. Bearing twelve children in sixteen years, Holly had four children in cloth diapers for years, yet she enjoyed her lifestyle.

She and her husband Craig taught the children to care for themselves, do household chores, share clothes and bedrooms, and eat simple, nutritious food. They entertained their children in groups, shared parenting tasks, kept a tight budget, and prayed and worshiped together. While Craig's two jobs helped him to avoid parental burnout, Holly became active in church groups in which she could interact with other women and return home refreshed.

Today, the ten children who have graduated from college are financially helping those two still in college. Five children are professionals; one is a member of the clergy. Holly's advice to harried mothers is, "Work hard, have patience, and pray a lot. Faith gives you strength."

FITTING THE BABY INTO THE OLDER FAMILY

Did you plan your children so that they would be born close together and could be playmates for each other? Maybe now you are pregnant with a baby you didn't plan who will be much younger than your other children. Find a playmate for this baby by calling up friends, relatives, local schools, and churches. Ask for the names of moms with small children. Most women will gladly let their children play at another mother's house.

A few children playing together in a designated spot, with a designated adult supervisor and for a designated time, is considered to be a play group. Ask mothers about joining an established play group or create your own. A church nursery may be a good spot for a play group.

Babysitting in your home provides playmates plus cash. Accept only the age children you want, or have your child cared for by a sitter who watches other children who are your child's age.

If you live in an isolated area, visit a playground, park, or family and let your child play with children there. When your child goes to school, invite his or her classmates to your house to play.

Don't overlook your older children. They'll probably lavish the baby with attention, leaving you time to work. A baby also teaches kids that healthy sexuality doesn't end at age twenty-five. Your children will learn about married love from you and your husband.

JUSTIFYING YOUR CHILD'S EXISTENCE

Today, certain people see children as consumers rather than builders of society. Parents with low incomes, more than two children, or babies they didn't plan are going to hear negative remarks about their children. They will also hear remarks if they are experiencing crises, which could get worse as a result of pregnancy. These crises include financial difficulty, health problems, emotional upheaval, or career changes.

Your child has a right to be! As Fran (Chapter Three) said, "I don't have to give people a reason for my child's existence." You don't have to, either.

Kris and her husband had four children, one mentally retarded and in special classes and another with a mild learning disability from brain damage at birth. When Kris became pregnant again, many "friends" said that five children was too many and dropped the family from their social calendar. Kris joked about their "evil eye" and made new friends who see her child as a worthwhile individual instead of a mistake.

If you're using family planning, this will probably be your only surprise baby. Family planning methods are fairly successful. Ask a doctor, nurse, or family planning counselor what might have gone wrong with your method. Learn from your mistake.

Artificial birth control is not the only effective option for controlling the size of your family. Modern natural family planning methods are reliable and safe. A hospital or doctor should be able to refer you to a natural family planning instructor.

Just because your method of family planning didn't work does not mean that your baby is a mistake. Many of us are the results of "mistakes" or "surprises," yet we enrich the world. That's how Arlene feels about her surprise baby. With their only child in the Army, she and her husband were planning a trip to Europe when Arlene became pregnant. "We signed on for the whole ride, not just the easy stuff," her husband said. Arlene says that raising this boy has been a joy.

More and More Surprises

You're going to have lots of surprises with your surprise baby! You'll discover new toys, birthing methods, weight gain requirements for pregnant moms, baby clothes, diapers, and mothering tactics. Your child will be unlike any other, and that will be a surprise. In fact, this child may one day be your greatest consolation. This is what happened to Rebecca (Chapter One), Sarah (Chapter Two), and Joyce (Chapter Three).

What if you wanted a child of one sex but your baby is of the opposite sex? Like most people, you'll probably accept and love the child you have. A child's sex doesn't guarantee a certain personality. Enjoy your child's individuality.

If you feel that you'll always resent your child, consider making an adoption plan. You needn't justify your plan. To invite another family to parent your child is to know your limits. If we all knew ourselves as well, we could make life easier for ourselves.

PROMISE OF A LIFETIME TOGETHER

If you see your baby as a gift, your life together will be bright and promising. Your child may not be coming at the most convenient time. Fitting your baby into your lifestyle may take unique adjustment. Ask for help. You may want to change the way you are doing some things. Get advice from others and take time for yourself. Love, patience, and the desire to parent your child will show you the way. A loved child can bring great rewards. Your love will help others love your child, too.

"The heart never 'gives up' a child. Adoption is a 'head decision.'"

—*M.P.N.*

Thinking About Adoption

You've already made one of the most important decisions of your life. You've decided to give birth. But have you decided to parent? Parenting right now might seem wrong for you. Answering the questions in Appendix G may reaffirm your adoption decision.

PARENTING BY RELATIVES, FRIENDS, OR ACQUAINTANCES

Parenting by relatives, friends, or acquaintances is not adoption. Simply ask a family to parent for you. You continue to make medical and legal decisions for your children, and you are legally and financially responsible for them. In time, you may be able to parent your children yourself.

Because she had difficulty parenting her large family, Eleanor asked her mother to parent one of her boys, who was close in age to some of her mother's sons—his uncles. After growing up between his mother's and grandmother's houses, the young man entered a business partnership with his uncles, whom he always considered brothers.

If you make someone your child's legal guardian, that person can make legal, medical, and educational decisions for your child. You may also make these decisions. Legal guardianship is wise if you will not be living near the parenting family.

However, you still retain all your parenting rights; you are legally free to parent your child yourself, at any time. A young teen, Katrin found it difficult to parent her infant so she made her married sister her baby's legal guardian and parent.

If you make a legal adoption plan with relatives, the relatives will legally become your baby's parents. Legal adoption can keep your pregnancy a secret while making your baby heir to your relative's estate.

LEGALIZING YOUR ADOPTION OR PARENTING ARRANGEMENT

Adoption choices and legal procedures are constantly changing. Contact a licensed adoption consultant, either an adoption attorney or a counselor at a licensed adoption agency or adoption service. This professional will help you make a legal plan, whether it is a private adoption, agency adoption, or other parenting arrangement including temporary parenting by relatives or friends. For your protection and that of your baby, all parties need to sign, in the presence of a witness (usually a notary), a legal, written parenting or adoption agreement. Neglecting these procedures may mean facing a sticky legal battle over parenting.

Find an adoption consultant by checking the phone book's adoption agency and adoption attorney listings. A child and family services agency may know adoption consultants. The Bar Association may list adoption attorneys. When you call a consultant, ask for additional referrals to others who arrange adoptions. Interview several consultants before choosing one.

Make an appointment with an adoption professional. Ask to see the person's credentials and license. Request a list of references or clients and call them. Were they pleased with the adoption professional? Why or why not? Ask the Better Business Bureau about consultants; the Bar Association about attorneys. Call the licensing agency (usually a governmental child and welfare agency) to be sure that the professional is licensed and in good standing.

If a consultant has no license or references or seems to be in legal or financial difficulty, find another consultant fast! If a consultant seems honest and professional, decide if that person offers the services you want and if you feel comfortable working with the individual. Appendix G lists some questions to consider before making a choice.

A good adoption consultant will be familiar with current adoption law. Together, the two of you will discuss parenting and adoption options, with you free to choose either one. If you want an unusual plan, the consultant should confirm the plan *in writing*. After your baby is born, your consultant will help you to rethink your decision, come to terms with any grief or mixed emotions, and finalize your plans. If you decide to parent, a consultant can suggest parenting classes.

ADOPTION IS A PERMANENT CHOICE

Adoption is a decision of the head, not of the heart—a loving, major decision, but a most difficult choice. Get as much information about adoption as you can, then think about it. Discuss the questions in Appendix G, and possibly some questions in Appendix F as well, with your adoption consultant. Whether you're married or single, you may realize that adoption is best for everyone.

In adoption, you're the birth mother and your baby's father is the birth father. The family who will parent your child is the adoptive family. An adoption plan is the plan you make with the adoptive family. Final adoption proceedings involve a very private hearing before a judge and the signing of final adoption papers. No one can call an adoption agency or court and get information on your baby's adoption. A consultant can answer questions about proceedings.

When you sign final adoption papers, you give the adoptive family the legal right to parent your child, forever. This assures that your baby has a permanent home and also ensures that your child will not be returned to your care.

It's very difficult to change a legal adoption arrangement unless a child is being abused. Child abuse is very unlikely, as adoption consultants carefully choose adoptive parents. In rare cases involving abuse, the child seldom goes back to the birth mother. Another family will probably adopt.

Adoption consultants have long lists of couples waiting to adopt. Many families will adopt children with special needs or terminal illnesses. Many couples have waited years for a child, and they will care for your baby well.

Ask a consultant what emotional, financial, age, and other requirements adoptive families must meet, what counseling they receive, and if they are studied before and after the adoption takes place. Choose a consultant who selects adoptive families carefully.

The more counseling you receive, and the more questions you ask and answers you get, the more certain you will be of adoption. Until you sign final adoption papers, usually weeks after your baby's birth, your baby is legally under your care. You'll have time to decide if adoption is right for you.

Don't be surprised if your parents, boyfriend, spouse, or friends try to talk you out of adoption. They'll have lots of reasons why you should parent, but are the reasons right for you? *You* are the one who will be parenting your baby. Can you or do you want to do it? *You* must make a parenting choice and you must be comfortable with it. Otherwise you may have regrets. Melody knew that adoption for her infant was right for her. With her husband in prison, she could barely parent her other two children.

Will Others Be Involved in Your Decision?

Just who has to be involved in an adoption decision, other than yourself, differs from area to area. An adoption consultant can tell you what your area requires. Everyone involved in making an adoption arrangement should receive adoption counseling. If you are under pressure from anyone to choose adoption, a judge may not approve the adoption.

In many places, no matter how young you are, your family may not legally plan the adoption of your baby, except in rare cases. They may advise you, but you must make the plan. If you're of legal age, you probably don't have to tell your family about your pregnancy or adoption plan. Andrea's and Kathleen's parents (see Chapter Two) still don't know that their daughters were pregnant.

Usually, the birth father, if you know who he is, or your husband (whether or not he is the actual father) will have to agree to the adoption. If no man claims legal responsibility for the child, then you are probably free to make your own plans.

You may face some sticky situations. Perhaps you are no longer in touch with the birth father, or don't ever want to see him again. You may be married, but pregnant because of an affair, as Pearl was, or you may have other concerns, all discussed in Appendix G. Discuss these situations with an adoption consultant. Usually, you can make plans that will put you at ease. Pearl, for example, reconciled with her husband, and the law considered him to be the child's legal father. Together they made an adoption plan.

If the birth father or his family or your family want to adopt your baby, they probably have to prove, in court, that they are financially secure, mentally stable, and morally sound, and that they would make good parents. If you have evidence to the contrary, tell a lawyer.

Having divorced her criminal husband, LeeAnn feared she'd abuse their three little children, so she chose one adoptive family to parent her infant and another for her two older children. A court agreed that these families, friends who attend the same church, would be better parents than LeeAnn's or her husband's relatives, who also wanted to adopt the children. LeeAnn keeps in touch with her family.

Choosing adoption means choosing love and making a decision for life. By talking over all your choices with a good adoption consultant, you can feel at peace with your decision. You will continue to love and think of your child forever. You have made a head decision, using all the love in your heart.

"Many babies are conceived unplanned, but no baby was ever adopted by accident."

—*An adoptive mother*

Making an Adoption Plan

Adoption comes in many packages. Sometimes the birth mother and adoptive family do not know each others' names and never meet. Their only contact is through an adoption consultant. Other times, the birth mother meets the adoptive family and may even visit her child following the adoption.

You must make a plan that meets your needs. You may want to forget this pregnancy or keep it a secret. Perhaps you want your child to bond well with the adoptive family with no interference from you. If so, you may not want to maintain contact with the adoptive family.

Perhaps you'd feel much more comfortable knowing your child's adoptive family and visiting as your child grows. You will feel as if you have a role in your child's life and not as if you are giving up your baby forever.

Appendix G will help you choose the type of adoption plan you want. After reading that, choose a consultant who can arrange this plan.

Maretta, Willa, and Tina had to search to make the adoption plans they wanted.

Maretta consulted several agencies before finding one that would allow her to meet the adoptive family, exchange photos, and visit her child.

Willa interviewed several couples, then had to choose again when her first choice couple adopted a baby from another agency.

When adoption regulations in Tina's state would not allow the birth mother and adoptive family to meet, she found an adoptive family through a friend's referral. Now she can visit her son as often as she likes.

ADOPTION CHOICES

You can help choose the adoptive family. The adoption consultant can select a family to meet your requirements in family size and makeup; ethnic, religious, educational, or social background; and so on. Or, the consultant may allow you to choose the adoptive family from several on file. You may be able to interview, either over the phone or in person, the adoptive families whose files you've selected. Then you will choose one family for your child. You may exchange identifying information with the family and even visit after your baby is adopted.

You can give your child a memento of yourself. You may compose a letter, tape-record a message, or make or select a special gift for your baby. You might ask that your child receive certain information at a certain age or that both of you maintain direct contact.

You can make an album or scrapbook of your baby's birth, take photos, and name your baby. Some adoptive parents use the name you've chosen as a middle name.

You may be able to see, hold, care for, and even breastfeed your baby in the hospital, if you wish. When you go home, others will parent your baby.

You and the adoptive family may not be in direct contact, as is the case with divorced Gracie and the family who adopted her child. Then the adoptive family may write letters about your baby's progress and send photos to the adoption consultant. The consultant will remove any identifying information and place the photos in your baby's file. You can request to see the file at any time. Gracie looks at her child's file a few times a year.

If you and your baby's father are on good terms, you may want him to participate in the adoption. Do what is comfortable for you both. If you and he disagree, your wishes will probably override his.

If you finalize an adoption, either the adoptive family or adoption consultant will pay your medical and counseling bills. Other expenses directly involved with the adoption, such as travel or shelter expenses, may also be paid for. An adoption consultant can tell you what bills, if any, are your responsibility. You should not be "paid for" your baby. This is illegal.

CONTACTING YOUR CHILD

In some adoption arrangements, neither you nor your child will know where the other lives. You will not be able to contact each other until your child reaches legal age and both of you consent to be found. Check the adoptive file to see if your child has written a letter asking for contact with you. If so, a court will open the file and let you find your child.

If you don't want your child to contact you, put your wishes *in writing* and ask your adoption consultant to place the letter in your baby's adoptive file. No one will be able to locate you. Should your child's health depend on vital medical information that only you can provide, you will be contacted very privately (your spouse, family, neighbors will not be involved).

If you do want to be found, write a letter to that effect and file it in the adoption file.

When Mary Jane's family wouldn't let her marry Dusty because of his religion, she had to make an adoption plan. However, later she and Dusty did marry and have two sons, but Mary Jane wanted to find her adopted daughter. At an adoption agency, she registered her desire for a reunion. Eight years later, her daughter, trying to find her birth mother, contacted the agency. Mary Jane and her daughter were reunited.

If you write a letter, then change your mind, call your adoption consultant and ask how you can insert a new letter into the adoption file. Follow the proper procedure. You may have to write a new letter, then have it notarized, witnessed, and sent by registered mail to the adoption consultant. The consultant will file the new letter and discard the old one.

If you will be in contact with your child as your child grows, you and the adoptive family will write up a contract. The contract will state how often you can contact and visit your child.

Many more families want to adopt babies than there are babies available. You can make a plan that suits you and find a consultant and family to go along with it. If you can't find anyone locally, tell a PREGNANCY AIDgency what you want. Ask the AIDgency to locate an agreeable consultant, and then to house you in that area so that you can make the adoption arrangement you want.

DEALING WITH GRIEF

Saying good-bye to the baby you've carried inside for nine months is very difficult. You'll probably feel intense grief and suddenly want to parent your baby. Because they will be aware that you feel so strongly, some doctors and nurses may discourage you from seeing, holding, or feeding your newborn. However, doing these things will give you a mental picture of your baby to remember and love. You'll know that choosing adoption is choosing love.

An adoption consultant can refer you to other birth mothers who have chosen adoption. Share your feelings with them, often. Learn how to handle and work through the grief, anger, resentment, and other strong emotions you may feel for months or longer. It's OK to cry. Feeling sad and hurt doesn't mean that you made the wrong decision. Many right decisions are painful ones. Once the emotional pain is gone, the rightness of your "head decision" will bring healing and peace.

Pregnant after being raped at a party, Opal, a quiet, gentle Native American teen-ager, asked an adoption agency to place her baby with a tribal family who lived off the reservation. Opal named and cared for her baby and made her a quilt and a teddy bear. She took photos for a scrapbook and wrote her infant a touching letter. When Opal found it too difficult to hand her baby to the adoptive couple, the agency asked her to visualize Jesus surrounded by children, then to see herself leaving her daughter in his lap while praying for her and the adoptive family. This helped Opal to express her grief and release her baby in her heart. After completing high school, Opal went on to college.

FOSTER CARE

Until you sign final adoption papers, your baby is still legally yours to parent. However, you will probably not take your baby home from the hospital. If the adoptive family does not have your child, a foster family will parent temporarily. When you sign the final adoption papers, usually when your baby is a few weeks old, the adoptive family will receive your child. It's best to finalize the adoption as quickly as possible.

You have the right to change your mind about adoption at any time until you sign the final adoption papers. If you have difficulty deciding about adoption, a lawyer or an adoption agency can arrange for your child to remain in foster care until you make up your mind.

A child in foster care does not have a permanent home and may move from one foster home to another. All these moves are traumatic, especially for children over eight months old. Leave your baby in foster care for no more than eight months, at most, before coming to a firm decision about adoption or parenting.

Meg and Heidi both had second thoughts when their babies were born. They placed their babies in foster care while they rethought adoption decisions.

Meg had chosen adoption as a way of denying her pregnancy, since only her boyfriend knew that she was pregnant at all. After four months of counseling, the couple decided that adoption was best.

Heidi had chosen adoption so that she could go to college. When she discovered that her state provided day care and financial aid for single mothers attending college, she took parenting courses and continued to attend college while parenting her child.

CHOOSING ADOPTION LATER

If you decide to parent, then change your mind after a few months of parenting, as LeeAnn (earlier in this chapter) and Terry (following) did, you can still make an adoption plan. It takes courage and a special love to admit you made a mistake. High schooler Terry knew that she was not a good mother to her six-month-old baby, whom she'd leave with her parents while she would date, party, and experiment with drugs. After making an adoption plan, she began to straighten out her life. Like Terry, you can find someone to parent your child. You and your child both deserve a future. Today Terry is a high school graduate with a job and a husband, and her baby is doing well in her adoptive home.

ADOPTION FOR SPECIAL GROUPS

In some countries, certain ethnic groups, races, or nationalities must follow special criteria in arranging adoptions. Tell your adoption consultant about your ethnic, racial, or national heritage and that of the birth father. If any special requirements apply to your baby, your consultant will know.

In the United States, for example, children with any percentage of Native American Indian blood must be adopted, if at all possible, by others of Native American Indian descent. These regulations insure that the child's Indian heritage will be preserved.

If special regulations apply, you may still be able to make any type of arrangement discussed in this chapter. However, the adoptive families you consider may have to possess ethnic, racial, or national characteristics that approximate those of your child. Many such families are eager to adopt, so you will have a good choice for your child. Choose a consultant who knows which regulations apply to you.

Marissa, an unmarried Native American, made an adoption plan under the guidelines set down by the Indian Child Welfare Act. Through a private agency that had done other Native American adoptions, Marissa requested that her child be the first child in the family and live in a rural setting. Marissa wanted her child's family to value education and to be of a certain religious denomination.

The agency contacted her tribe, which had no adoptive families within the tribe. The agency then identified five nontribal Native American families who met Marissa's requirements. Marissa read a file on each family and chose the family she liked best. The family annually updates the agency's file on Marissa's baby. Letters and photos show Marissa how her child is maturing.

MOVING ON

Whether or not you have contact with the adoptive family, you'll never forget your baby. When you remember, don't deny your feelings. Work through them. It's natural to regret not being able to raise your baby. It's also natural to feel relieved, and possibly guilty, about choosing adoption.

Remember, you are choosing adoption because it is the best choice for both you and your baby at this time of your lives. In Robert Frost's famous poem *The Road Not Taken*, the traveler stands at a fork in the road, wondering which road to take. After starting down one road, the traveler wonders about the other. Where would it have gone? Yet the road now taken is "fair," as was the other. Adoption isn't "better" than parenting, or vice versa. Both are fine choices. While you may wonder what might have been had you chosen differently, you have certainly chosen something good.

Chapter Six

GETTING OVER SEXUAL TRAUMAS

"No woman is born wearing an 'Open House' sign."

—M.P.N.

Dealing With Sexual Violence

Sexual violence leaves you feeling dirty, used, guilty, and shameful. Abused physically and emotionally, your very soul has been violated. If you are a victim of sexual trauma, you will need to work through your feelings and learn how to prevent a recurrence of that kind of violence.

CHILDHOOD MOLESTATION

According to recent studies, as many as one in three adult women may have been sexually molested, often frequently, as children. Someone you trusted may have molested you. Molestation can involve touching, fondling, or unclothing, and may escalate into intercourse. You may have also been physically or emotionally abused or neglected.

You may have felt molested if, as a young child, you were treated medically, especially in the genital or rectal area. If your relationship with your parents, especially your father, was poor at that time, you may have subconsciously felt sexually damaged, worthless, and abandoned. Now, you may have addictions or be insecure in relationships with men.

Sexual molestation involves control by others stronger than you. You may still let others decide for you, or you may lash back in an effort to take control. For this pregnancy, do what is best for you and your baby, no matter what others are telling you. Don't do what they say because they say it, or do the opposite to show that you, and not they, are in control. The damaged, controlled, abused child in you can become a sensitive, capable woman as you plan for your baby.

RAPE

Every woman fears rape. If you are a victim of this violent, degrading crime, you can't bury the memory. News of your pregnancy might devastate others; hiding your secret devastates you. You may want to lie, abort your baby, run away, or kill yourself. These feelings may seem especially overpowering if two or more men took turns violating you, as happened to Shannie (refer to Chapter Three).

Find a counselor who will help you voice your strong, conflicting emotions and release your guilt and shame. You are a *victim*. You are *not* responsible for your own sexual assault.

Suppose the man who assaulted you is emotionally or mentally ill due to addiction, abuse, genetic makeup, illness, or other reasons. Suppose he was parented poorly or not at all. You are not responsible for these conditions.

What if the assailant has no addictions or emotional problems? A mentally stable man can *always* control himself sexually, even on a date. "I just couldn't control myself" should be "I just *wouldn't* control myself." If a policeman were in the next room, the assaulting man would have "controlled himself."

Nothing gives a man, even a husband, the right to enter a woman's body without her express permission. If someone (even a friend or relative) were to barge into another person's home without being invited in, the homeowner would feel violated. How much more violated a woman feels if her body is entered without her permission!

You aren't responsible for assault, but you are responsible for dealing with your feelings about it. Vent your hatred, anger, and repulsion. Know where you hurt. The hardest person you'll have to deal with may be yourself.

> *After a stranger beat and raped her, Ina refused her family's pressure to abort and told her fiancé. During a Christmas Eve service, he thought of Joseph, who stood by his wife Mary and raised Jesus, whom he had not fathered. Ina's fiancé married Ina. Together they are raising Ina's daughter as their own child.*

Emotional Turmoil

If you are a victim of sexual assault, you may feel no emotion when you learn you're pregnant. Numbness eventually becomes repulsion, anger, and despair. Your disgust for the rapist may transfer to your baby. Yet your baby did not assault you or ask to be conceived. Your baby is a victim, too.

Many people mistakenly believe that continuing your pregnancy will torture you with memories of the rape. Actually, with counseling, going through the pregnancy and birth will help you work through hatred and repulsion. Eventually, you will feel good about yourself for giving your baby a future. Later in this chapter you'll learn how to find a sympathetic counselor for sexual trauma.

Maybe you want to keep your pregnancy a secret. You may feel that you will never be comfortable parenting your baby. You know that adoption will give your baby a family, so that is always a choice, as it was for Opal (Chapter Five). However, you may decide to parent your baby as Bonnie (Chapter Seven) and Shannie (Chapter Three) did.

INCEST

Incest is rape within the family. If you are an incest victim, the preceding discussion will help you, but you have much additional confusion to sort through.

Incest leaves unique emotional scars. You may love the incestuous family member yet hate him for what he does. Pregnancy makes you wonder if your baby will be deformed or if the police will arrest the abuser.

Most children conceived through incest are normal. If your baby was fathered by a relative who is related to you by your mother's remarriage, your child's risk of abnormality is no greater than any other child's would be. If you are a blood relative of the sexual abuser, your child has a 55 percent to 85 percent chance of being normal. If your child does have special needs or a fatal condition, refer to Chapter Seven.

Hiding incest helps no one. While the community need not know, your family should know about incest (and possibly does). Incest can go on for generations and may involve other victims in your family. You may almost think that incest is normal. It's not.

In a normal family, only the husband and wife engage in intercourse or other sexual actions. Fathers and daughters, mothers and sons, brothers and sisters, and other relatives limit body contact to occasional, spontaneous, brief, loving hugs and kisses. This *never* proceeds to fondling, unclothing, and beyond. Incestuous family members see each other as objects of sexual exploration and enjoyment. You'll feel, rightly, that the incestuous person is more interested in you sexually than in the real, feeling you.

Family members may choose not to believe that incest is going on. Glenda's mother chose not to believe Glenda's claims of incest, and Luciana was afraid to tell her mother about her stepfather's sexual abuse.

Although Glenda's father sexually abused her for thirteen years, her mother chose to believe that Glenda was "dreaming." Even when her husband got Glenda pregnant at fifteen, and then had a vasectomy, Glenda's mother believed her daughter's story that she had been raped while babysitting. At the family's insistence, Glenda made an adoption plan, and the incest continued until Glenda left home at the age of eighteen. Glenda has had years of counseling to deal with the incest. She has also visited her daughter and adoptive family.

Luciana never told her mother about her stepfather's sexual abuse, begun when she was six. When Luciana became pregnant at eleven, her mother thought that she had been sexually active, and her stepfather said, "We've got to show her all our love." The family adopted Luciana's baby boy. Only later, when Luciana's mother threatened divorce if her husband didn't stop having affairs, did he admit, "That boy you love so much is mine." When Luciana acknowledged the incest, her shocked mother refused to allow her husband into their living quarters. After learning job skills, she got a divorce and moved out, taking Luciana and her son with her.

Stopping Incest

Families allow incest to continue by denying or hiding it. Family members may swear that they will see that the incest stops if you lie about the pregnancy or abort. This promise won't work. A family caught in incest addiction is almost always powerless to stop without professional help. In order to stop the incest, you will probably have to tell someone outside your family about it. Talk to someone immediately. Choose a professional such as a member of the clergy, social worker, teacher, guidance counselor, or PREGNANCY AIDgency volunteer.

A professional can help each family member vent emotional pain and heal. Victims need to learn appropriate ways to seek help. Abusers need to overcome incest and other addictions. People who enable incest to continue need to face their denial.

A professional counselor will embarrass no one. Unless the family presses charges, no one will go to jail. No one will be judged or made to feel guilty. Problems discussed in a counselor's office remain confidential.

If your family won't go for counseling, go by yourself. By concealing your pregnancy and possibly relocating elsewhere, you and your baby can be safe. If you tell a child welfare agency about your home situation, you can probably be moved into foster care if you are a minor. If you're an adult, you can leave home by using government aid. You may consider adoption for your baby.

If you return home, you'll want to devise ways to stop the incest and keep your baby safe if you'll be parenting. You'll also have to learn appropriate ways of parenting and dealing sexually with your child. A counselor can help you. Consider, however, that it is wiser for you and your baby to leave a home where incest continues than to stay there and risk future abuse.

If you have experienced sexual violence, you need much emotional healing. You are a victim, and so is your baby. Both you and your child are worthwhile human beings who deserve respect, understanding, and help. Reach out for the help you need.

"The Streets taught me to trust no one, 'love don't love nobody' . . . .
I now see that my street learnings are not all that I want to base my life on."

— *"Vibrant," a former prostitute*

Overcoming Sexual Pressure

Do you make your own decisions? Do you indulge in a lifestyle that controls you? Does this control make it difficult for you to give birth to your baby? It's time to evaluate just how much control you have over your life.

SEXUAL ADDICTION

Six percent of United States citizens crave sex and frequently have multiple partners. They can't stop this behavior. These people are sex addicts. Are you one also?

Society misunderstands sexual addiction. Yes, people view indecent phone calls, exhibitionism, rape, incest, and child molestation as perversions. However, you may have multiple partners and one-night stands, or you may participate regularly in group sex. People may consider you foolish for risking AIDS, but they probably don't think that you need help. However, you might actually be unable to control your bed hopping. If you crave sexual experience, but then hate yourself for your excess, you are battling a sexual addiction.

Although sex addicts can come from any type of background, their family backgrounds often reveal neglect, alcoholism, drug addiction, or abuse (whether physical, emotional, or sexual). You're probably a sex addict if you can't stop your sexual behavior, no matter what it is. You may have other addictions, too.

Your behavior is an addiction if it follows the SAFE formula, developed by Dr. Patrick Carnes, a pioneer in the field of sexual addiction. The formula is as follows:

S— Your behavior is a *Secret*. You'd be ashamed to let the public know of this behavior.

A— Your behavior is *Abusive*. You harm, manipulate, or degrade yourself or others.

F— The behavior helps you avoid painful *Feelings* or makes you feel better or feel worse.

E— Your behavior is *Empty* of a caring, committed relationship to the people involved with your behavior.

If you see yourself in the SAFE formula, you're probably a sex addict. If pregnancy is the result, it is extra frightening. It may make public your addiction and bring rejection, or it may keep you from continuing your addiction—a scary thought. At the same time, pregnancy might bring an end to your addiction, and you desperately want to control sex and feel worthwhile and lovable again.

You cannot stop an addiction to sex on your own. You need the support of caring individuals, some of whom have been where you are now, to help you. These people will help you see that you *are* a worthwhile person. People *can* accept you. Sex need *not* be the most important part of your life. A self-help group for sexual addiction or other addictive behavior, counselor, or member of the clergy may help you overcome your addiction. A helpline, hotline, or mental health agency can make a referral. You'll learn why you're an addict, how to deal with your past, and how to control your behavior.

When you control your sexual addiction, you can make plans for your baby. A PREGNANCY AIDgency will help you. By overcoming sexual addiction now, you are making a good future for your baby and for yourself.

Jayne's alcoholic mother and workaholic father gave her a strict moral upbringing and lots of material goods, but little personal attention. In college, she became sexually active with two men and began to question her faith. Having had one abortion, which depressed her, she bore a child by a third man even though he, like her second lover, wanted her to abort. Over the next years, she experienced a series of one-night stands, a brief marriage, and suicidal thoughts. She also underwent psychiatric counseling, was involved with a bizarre religious cult, and made periodic trips to mental institutions.

Eventually, Jayne began to attend a more conventional prayer group, whose members helped her deal with her past and reclaim her faith. Finally, she joined a growing religious community, whose founder had been devastated by sexual ex-

cess, atheism, and abortion. Jayne married a community member, who adopted her daughter as well as another child. Both Jayne and her husband endured crises and worked on their problems individually, together, and with counselors. Still working to heal past wounds, Jayne and her husband have a deep faith and are happy.

PROSTITUTION

If you're a prostitute, you are viewed as living on the margin of society. You may find it awkward or difficult to reach out for help with your pregnancy.

Many pregnant prostitutes, call girls, and escorts want to have their babies. You probably know some who have done so. They may be parenting their children or they may have chosen adoption. There is much that is bitter, tarnished, and hateful in prostitution. But your baby is grace, innocent beauty, and a pure beginning.

If you're independently employed, you may need government assistance or another job to support you for a time. On the other hand, a pimp or madam may pressure you to abort so that you can keep working. You may be both afraid of and in love with a pimp. Some pimps and madams have connections to organized crime. Your life may be in danger if you attempt to continue your pregnancy or run away. What sort of pressure are you under? Do you foresee any pressure?

Insecurity and fear may keep you from seeking help. You should fight thoughts such as: "I can't do any work but prostitution." "If people know my past, they'll reject me." "I can't live in poverty." "I have no skills." "I don't know how to act in straight society." "I'm dumb." "I don't want to be bored." "I use drugs, and no one will want to help me." "I have AIDS or VD so what's the use of having my baby?" "My pimp abuses me, but he loves me. I couldn't get any other man, anyway."

The right counselors will not reject you. Call a PREGNANCY AIDgency, women's shelter, rape crisis center, or women's resource center for help. A shelter for battered women is a safe haven. A PREGNANCY AIDgency can move you anywhere in the country (or even out of it) so that you will be safe.

You may have experienced rape, incest, neglect, sexual molestation, or physical or emotional abuse, which has left many emotional scars. You may have problems that need treatment such as a disease, AIDS, addictions, a pressuring boyfriend, or some other fear. If you had a poor upbringing, you may need to learn parenting skills, money management, social graces, and job skills. You may even decide to leave prostitution but wonder if you can succeed socially and financially in "straight society." Find a good counselor, following the guidelines later in this chapter, and share your concerns. You can certainly make a new life for yourself, with new skills and new friends, if you believe in yourself and are willing to try.

A self-employed prostitute, Yvonne's plan of becoming pregnant to keep her boyfriend didn't work. She left prostitution and went into a shelter for homeless women. With the help of a counseling agency, she learned secretarial skills and rented an apartment. She and another woman took turns babysitting each other's children while each worked. Yvonne is proud of her success.

YOU HAVE FREEDOM

If you feel enslaved to a lifestyle, you still have some freedom.

- Freedom to overcome a lifestyle.
- Freedom to think.
- Freedom to seek help.
- Freedom to give birth to your baby.
- Freedom to change yourself.

Find a friend, a counselor, and possibly a self-help group to help you. Together, you can heal your emotional wounds, leave the past behind you, and build a promising future.

"A woman is much more than the sum total of her body parts."

—*M.P.N.*

Creating a New You

Women are much more than sexual beings. If a sexual relationship lacks love, respect, and caring, and sometimes even brings physical harm, a woman may feel used. You can be totally unaware that sexual trauma has made you view yourself and the world differently. If you don't heal emotionally, your damaged self-image may cause you to make poor decisions in many areas of life.

Fiona was raised in an abusive, unsupportive home. The only thing she liked about herself was her virginity. While in graduate school, Fiona was cleaning up after a college function when Steve, a classmate of another race, violently attacked and raped her, destroying her treasured virginity. Fiona loathed herself. Now what did she have to offer a husband?

Months later, another classmate Paul, whom Fiona hated and knew to be an unsavory, immoral character, asked Fiona for a date. She felt undeserving of anyone better, so she accepted. Because Fiona considered her raped body no longer worthy of love, respect, or dignity, she let Paul repeatedly fondle and rape her on several dates. When Fiona became pregnant, Paul called her "a tramp." Then he offered to marry her.

Paul made Fiona quit school, then quit himself. They lived in poverty, with Paul drinking heavily. Two months after their son was born, a drunken Paul tried to choke and rape Fiona, who called the police. Saying he wasn't even sure the baby was his, Paul sent Fiona home to her parents. Eventually the marriage was annulled. Fiona's son developed discipline problems and eventually alcoholism, and she questioned whether she should have made an adoption plan for her child.

Fiona has worked many jobs and had many affairs, some involving emotional abuse. Hospitalized several times for mental illness, she has been in psychological counseling for over thirty years. Fiona writes, "For forty years I have been haunted by a sense of being dirty, used, contaminated, and unfit to associate with decent people. I have always associated sex with hate and violence and being dominated and humiliated. I have never experienced sex as love."

Fiona used to repeatedly call a PREGNANCY AIDgency hotline just to listen to the recording which began, *"You are a person of worth and dignity."* She is still trying to believe that about herself.

Fiona's story indicates the need to heal the wounds of sexual trauma. Burying wounds and feeling shame when you are the victim causes deeper wounds and loss of self-esteem. With little self-esteem, you continue to form traumatic relationships, as Fiona did.

Sexual trauma includes molestation, rape, incest, sexual addiction, prostitution, and group sex, which are all discussed earlier in this chapter. It also results from sexually transmitted diseases, AIDS, abortion, and physically damaging sexual acts. If you have been a victim of any of these things, a doctor can treat you medically, but you need counseling to resolve the bitterness you feel toward yourself and others.

MENTAL TRAUMA

A child can be sexually traumatized emotionally while never being touched physically. Some families or peer groups push girls into early dating. The media often imply that being sexually tantalizing and having intercourse are important ways to prove that you're mature.

Do you have sex because "everybody's doing it"? Everybody's not! According to the United States National Center for Health Statistics, at least 17 percent of all women are virgins at marriage, and at least 10 percent of all unmarried women have never had intercourse by age forty-four. Moreover, many of those who have been sexually active actually have intercourse very infrequently. Yes, having sex can be enjoyable and fun, but don't do it just because "everybody's doing it." How do you feel about it? It's OK to say "No," "Not yet," or "Not with you." Remember, having sex doesn't indicate maturity, creativity, wit, intelligence, or love. Baboons have sex frequently, but would you want to date a baboon? (Maybe you've already dated one!)

Maybe you feel you "owe" your date sex. You don't! Would you visit a friend and demand dinner if you weren't asked to eat? A friend doesn't owe you dinner because you visit. You don't owe a man sex because he dates you. If he feels that way, let him date somebody else.

You may feel that you have to have sex to "hold on to" your man. If you don't deliver, he'll find someone else. Why not let a man go if he's dating you only for sex? Suppose you contracted an illness or sustained an injury and couldn't perform. Where would this man's "love" be then?

Pregnancy can add more trauma to your relationship. If your lover is standing by you, encouraging you to give birth, you're fortunate. This will decrease your stress.

However, pregnancy may make your lover distant or angry, or he may pressure you to get an abortion. He might even fade out of the picture. All the promises your lover made may dissolve once you're pregnant. Your lover may say he wants you to abort because it's "best for you," but maybe he really feels it's best for him. Maybe he wants you to be sexually available. Maybe he wants no responsibility for the baby. If this is the case, having your baby might mean losing your man. But is someone like this worth keeping?

Reevaluate your relationship. Did you allow yourself to be used? Were you looking for a man—any man—to replace the love you never had from a father? Did you jump into a relationship to avoid dealing with a recent hurt? Did you choose a man who prizes a sexually available, alluring body above everything else? Did you overlook warning signs and hints of your lover's true character? What can you learn from this experience so that you don't repeat it?

Nikki had one disastrous sexual relationship and wanted no more. Jackie was a virgin until she met Bruce. Nikki became pregnant when a stranger, whom she was trying to comfort after a family tragedy, pressured her into intercourse. Jackie consented to intercourse to snare about-to-be-divorced Bruce, who said he'd never marry again unless he "had to." Abandoned by their lovers to deal with their pregnancies, Jackie and Nikki worked through tumultuous emotions and despair to give birth. Nikki is parenting her son; Jackie chose a family she knew to adopt her daughter. Both women now speak to teens and urge them to control their sexuality.

SECONDARY VIRGINITY

You can learn from your mistakes. If you have made foolish choices regarding sex and relationships and want to stop that kind of behavior, why not claim "secondary virginity"? Secondary virgins are women who have been sexually active but who have now chosen to keep sex out of casual relationships. They reclaim virginity because they don't "owe" a man sex. Secondary virgins wait to "have sex" until a man makes a permanent commitment, often marriage.

Secondary virginity is not "holding off the goodies" or "being a prude." It's protecting yourself from possible emotional harm, pregnancy, or disease.

Any man can be on good behavior to get you in bed. But what is this guy *really* like? Keep intense sexual activity out of the relationship, and you'll talk and share more. You'll get to *know* someone, who will get to know *you*. A man should love you for yourself. You should love the real man, not a fantasy.

When you've been sexually active, it's hard to change, but you can do it! Keep your clothes on! Ask a date to take you home if things start getting unbuttoned. If you don't want to have intercourse, staying dressed works.

Some men will ask for a sexual relationship. They might drop you if they're ready but you're not; however, others will be glad to wait until you are ready. Which type of man would you rather date?

Maybe you think you don't deserve someone who respects your wishes in a relationship. Why do you feel this way? Perhaps you should speak to a counselor or member of the clergy. With help, you will learn to be strong in your convictions and realize that you should let your own values direct your behavior and not cave in to pressure from someone else.

If you hate to keep attracting men who push you into having sex, you may be looking in the wrong places for dates. Look beyond the local bar or disco and reconsider your neighbor, fellow employee, or classmate. Or look at the men whom you frequently meet in a civic, ecological, religious, literary, political, self-help, or humanitarian group.

Also consider changing your image of the perfect male date. Often the most compassionate and interesting men are not the most physically attractive or socially graceful. Give a shy, less handsome man a chance. You may find someone special.

To find the right man you may have to make some changes, too. Maybe the way you flirt or dress attracts men who want women who are easy to get into bed. If you tone down your flirtations and the way you dress, you might attract a less aggressive male.

Maybe you'll meet a man who wants to marry a woman who is willing to wait to have intercourse until marriage. If he doesn't ask you for intercourse, don't suggest it yourself. If you are sexually aggressive with a man who values his own virginity, you may scare away a good friend and a potential partner.

Deeply in love with Arthur, Martha initiated intercourse. Upset because he had compromised his own values and lost his virginity before his marriage, Arthur immediately dropped Martha. Eventually he married Martha's best friend. She and Arthur now have a child. Martha is still looking for "Mr. Right."

If you want to get married someday, you, too, may be looking for "Mr. Right." Perhaps you think you've found him. Talk over what you will be sharing together—meals, sex, home, finances, children, thoughts, values, hobbies, and religion. Will you be able to adjust to each other? Will this man love and respect you, or does he have problems that could be difficult to handle in a marriage? Appendix F has many questions to consider when you're facing the decision to marry.

FINDING A COUNSELOR

Unless they have personally experienced sexual trauma, few people can understand its agony. You probably do not understand your own depth of pain and confusion. You need someone who will help you deal with having your baby while you work to uncover and address all your repressed emotions.

A PREGNANCY AIDgency is the best place to look for help. Every volunteer can help plan for your future and your baby. Many volunteers are also extremely sensitive to victims of sexual trauma. Some will spend much time with you as you confront and work through your pain. If you meet a volunteer who seems unfeeling, casual, judgmental, or incompetent, or who is simply a busybody, ask to speak to the AIDgency director. Tell her your situation and request another volunteer, or go to another PREGNANCY AIDgency, or ask an AIDgency to refer you to professional or other help.

Professional help can include social workers, psychologists, and members of the clergy who are trained to deal with victims of sexual trauma. You may find compassionate counselors at rape crisis centers, child abuse centers, women's shelters, and drug and alcohol abuse clinics. The counselor must be sympathetic toward your decision to have your baby. One who thinks you should abort will only add stress to your life.

You may be able to find compassionate counselors through referrals from area prayer groups, places of worship, hotlines, self-help anonymous groups for various addictions including sexual addiction, and after-abortion helplines (check the classified ads or call a local pro-life group). Also call some of the national hotlines in Appendix H for referral to local agencies that might have counselors for you.

If you find an insensitive counselor, keep looking. A good counselor will help you understand that both you and your baby are persons of worth and dignity. You will learn to recognize hurts, deal with them, and love yourself.

LET GO OF THE PAST AND EMBRACE THE FUTURE

Sexual trauma leaves you feeling victimized and defiled. You may hate yourself and think you deserve the pain. Holding on to bitter memories enslaves you to the past. Sure, you can't change what's happened. But you can change yourself and you can change your future.

You need to see yourself as a worthwhile person who deserves happiness. The past is done. Even if you willingly consented to sexual activity, you are still a victim of pressures on you to have intercourse. These pressures can come from others or from your own reasons why you thought you had to have intercourse. Since you never foresaw where your activity would lead, you should stop punishing yourself for your actions or their consequences. Forgive yourself so you can love yourself.

A good counselor will help you to release bitterness toward and forgive those who assaulted or victimized you. Then you will accept your own victimization.

Forgiveness does not mean justifying the evil done to you. It means giving up your right to demand revenge. Your assailants are responsible for their behavior and deserve punishment. Born innocent children, they were damaged by human faults, emotional wounds, and mistaken, corrupt beliefs. They are victims of poor upbringing, wrong choices, hormonal or chemical imbalances, or past experiences. Enjoying evil and not knowing good, your assailants are victims, too. Forgiveness means recognizing that fact.

At some point, you may want to tell these people that you forgive them. If this is not possible, or is too painful, you might picture your assailants in your mind and mentally voice your forgiveness to them.

Forgiving those who harmed you may not change them, but it will change you. Bitterness picks at the scab of sexual trauma. Forgiveness slowly heals the festering wound. Yes, you'll always have a scar, but you need not always have pain. Talk to a counselor today. You are a person of worth and dignity. You deserve to feel joy. Today can be the first day of your healing.

Chapter Seven

PAINFUL CIRCUMSTANCES

*"Death is the peak of a life-wave, and so is birth.
Death and birth are one."*

—*Abba Hillel Silver*

Facing Your Own Death

You may be facing terminal illness and be pregnant. It may be that your illness was discovered after your pregnancy began, or that you were ill and then became pregnant. Possibly your doctor has told you that there is a small chance that you could die during delivery. If you are facing death, either because of this pregnancy or otherwise, your emotions may be far worse than any you've experienced before. You are likely to experience the stages of loss that were first defined by Elisabeth Kubler-Ross in her now classic book *On Death and Dying*.

An immediate reaction may be either calm outward acceptance or total hysteria. This coping mechanism gives way to shock and denial, then fear and dread, worry and anxiety. Soon you'll feel angry, bitter, helpless, or out of control. You'll begin to bargain with God and your medical team. Eventually you'll come to accept your diagnosis. As you begin to heal emotionally, you'll be able to make decisions.

TERMINAL ILLNESS

If your illness really is terminal, ending your pregnancy won't save your life, although it may prolong it. Ask your doctor to be honest. Request statistics and probabilities on your life expectancy if you continue the pregnancy and if you end it. Find out if an early delivery of your baby might give you both a better chance of survival. If you don't believe your doctor, get several other opinions. Weigh the information and decide what to do. You may want to have your baby, no matter what the diagnosis.

If you really are facing death, you'll need counseling to help you deal with your conflicting thoughts and emotions. Some doctors and clergy make good counselors for the dying; many do not. If possible, contact a hospice.

Not to be confused with a hospital, a hospice cares for and counsels terminally ill individuals and their families. A hospice usually accepts only those patients who have a short time to live and for whom further treatment would be useless. With hospice care, you will probably continue to live at home, except for when you give birth or experience any pregnancy problems that require hospitalization. You'll receive pain medication and be kept comfortable, but your illness won't be treated aggressively unless doing so would give your baby a better chance of survival. Hospice workers will help you and your family accept death, and you will probably die at home.

Pregnancy Help

Well-meaning relatives, friends, and professionals may be pressuring you to end your pregnancy to prolong your life. Perhaps they are worried that medications and treatments may have harmed your baby. On the other hand, you may want to give birth because you feel your baby deserves a chance.

Discuss pressures and concerns with a confidant or a PREGNANCY AIDgency volunteer. Request treatments or medications that are safer for your baby. Tell your doctors, your family, and your friends that you are going to have your baby and that you are hoping for their love and support.

As much as you are able, make choices about your child's future. Will your partner, friends, or relatives parent your child? Will the person who is parenting need the help of a baby sitter, nanny, or household helper? Are you well enough to interview applicants and hire one? Would you prefer an adoptive family? Write down or tape-record any definite ideas about how you would like your child to be raised. Ask the parenting person to assure that your wishes will be met. Arranging details will make you feel more secure about your baby's future.

> During the sixth month of Lily's fifth pregnancy, doctors discovered ovarian cancer. Lily refused further surgery until doctors could perform a Cesarean section and deliver a living baby. By the time of the C-section, the cancer had spread drastically. Having spoken to her husband about parenting arrangements, Lily died two weeks after giving birth. Community members, church friends, and relatives gave much assistance to Lily's family. The older children babysat the younger. Another mother watched the baby while Lily's husband was at work. The family managed the best they could.

Perhaps you'd like to write a letter or booklet or tape-record a conversation for your child, like Rae did (Chapter Four). If you need help with this, ask a confidant or hospice volunteer.

Make a list of the ways people can help you, and have it printed at a local copy shop. Hand out this list to those who care. Wendy Bergren included these items on her list: cook a dinner, pray, tell me jokes, bake and freeze homemade pastries, and babysit. (See Appendix I for how to obtain a copy of Wendy's list.) By making a list, you'll receive the help you need.

Do you have any unfinished business? Do you need to write a will? Should you mend a relationship with someone? With God? Work on addressing these responsibilities now.

View your life realistically. Make a list of your successes and achievements—the bright spots. Speak about your fears and angers to God and to those who can offer comfort and direction. Rejoice in your baby's life. Strive for a peace that will remain until death.

Suppose You Die First?

Suppose you die before the baby is born? Modern technology *may* be able to keep your body alive until your baby's birth. If you want your baby to live, put your desire into writing *now* and file it with a lawyer.

> *When pregnant Helen suffered total brain death during an operation to remove a brain tumor, her live-in lover Yates remembered her last words, "You take care of the baby." Despite objections from Helen's mother, he fought a legal battle to keep Helen's body alive for almost two months until her baby was mature enough to be born and live. Yates's married sister is raising the baby while Yates remains the proud and loving father. The child is also in touch with Helen's parents.*

UTERINE AND CERVICAL CANCER

Pregnancy *may* cause your death if you have an advanced, untreated case of uterine or cervical cancer. Carrying your baby to term *may* give the cancer enough time to spread to other internal organs and endanger your life. However, if the cancer is not advanced and is under treatment, it may be possible for you to give birth without severely threatening your life. For example, some doctors will treat the cancer, deliver your baby early by Cesarean section, and then administer more aggressive treatments. If you have these cancers, consult several doctors so that you can obtain and consider different treatment options before making any decisions. You may be willing to risk death in order to give your baby a chance.

> *Vera and Zita had uterine cancer and wanted their unborn babies to live. Under her doctor's close supervision, Vera (Chapter Three) continued her pregnancy and gave birth early by Cesarean section before undergoing surgery for the cancer. Both she and her teenaged son are healthy today. Zita, a doctor, knew that her very malignant uterine cancer would kill her if doctors did not remove her uterus. However, removing her uterus would kill her baby. A very prayerful woman, Zita chose to continue the pregnancy and died two weeks after the birth of her healthy fourth child.*

ECTOPIC PREGNANCY

An ectopic pregnancy is often life threatening. In 95 percent of ectopic pregnancies, the baby is growing in a Fallopian tube. The Fallopian tube leads from the ovary, where the egg is released, to the uterus, where babies normally develop. At this time, doctors can't safely transplant the baby to the uterus. Doctors must remove the baby before the growing infant bursts the tube, causes internal bleeding, and dies. If a rupture occurs, the mother might die.

The remaining 5 percent of ectopic pregnancies occur in the ovary, cervix, or abdominal cavity. A baby growing in the abdominal cavity has a small chance of growing to nearly full term and being born alive.

If you have cramping, bleeding, or a pain or lump in your side during the first two months of pregnancy, ask your doctor to test for an ectopic pregnancy. Otherwise, you could be in serious danger.

Despite Lynn's severe cramps, excessive blood loss, two fainting spells, and a lump in her side, her doctor never diagnosed ectopic pregnancy. Instead, once Lynn's pregnancy test registered negative, the physician scheduled a routine operation to empty her womb. Overhearing Lynn's symptoms, another doctor examined Lynn and discovered a ruptured ectopic pregnancy that could have killed Lynn or destroyed her entire reproductive system. A quick operation saved Lynn, who went on to have other children (see Lynn's story in Chapter Two).

OTHER CONDITIONS

Other than ectopic pregnancy and some cases of advanced, untreated uterine or cervical cancers, modern medicine can manage most health conditions, including diabetes, heart disease, kidney disease, treated cancers, leukemia, multiple sclerosis, ostomies, and lupus, so that you can give birth without dying from the pregnancy. Chapter Four contains many stories of women with health problems who safely gave birth. In addition, repeat Cesarean section is much safer than it was thought to be. Irene has had eight Cesarean births and knows of a woman who has had thirteen.

If you're told that your pregnancy will cause your death, ask your doctors the questions in Appendix E. You may have additional questions. You'll want to know the *exact* reasons why your doctors predict death, the probability of your dying, and how your doctors can minimize or eliminate the risk. Request facts and literature on your condition. Read about what you are facing and think about your doctors' suggestions. Chapters Three and Four will give you additional guidelines. Dire consequences may be only a slight possibility. Good medical treatment might greatly increase your chances for a safe pregnancy.

You are the one who wants to have your baby. *You* make the final decisions. If you're insistent, your doctors are likely to go along with your wishes. If some doctors won't treat you, find others who will.

OVERCOMING SUICIDAL TENDENCIES

If your situation has led you to think about suicide, seek counseling at once! Don't assume that those around you "know" or "sense" what you are planning and would stop you if they cared. Most people don't "sense" that someone is planning suicide, nor do they take seriously any mention of suicide. People will either be angry with you for mentioning it, or they will ignore you. They may joke about suicide or even dare you to do it! These attitudes will upset you more. Get help!

Immediately call either a suicide prevention hotline, the local police, or a hospital, or call a national twenty-four-hour, toll-free hotline (some numbers are listed in Appendix H). Counselors will help you deal with your immediate disturbing thoughts. They will *not* send someone to whisk you away to the nearest psychiatric hospital or police station. If you want to speak to someone in person, ask that someone be sent to you. If you want to go to a hospital, say so.

Also call a PREGNANCY AIDgency twenty-four-hour hotline (see Appendix H) to learn what pregnancy help is available. A local AIDgency may be able to locate a professional counselor to help you, perhaps with no fee.

Problems Have Solutions

Every problem *does* have a solution that you *can* handle. You have more strength, talent, and hope than you know. You can make good choices, learn to cope with life, find joy in living, and believe in yourself. You can find people who really care.

Make yourself six promises.

1. For your own sake, promise yourself that you won't act on your thoughts of suicide for at least a year.
2. Determine to call both a PREGNANCY AIDgency and a suicide hotline for help *today, now.*
3. Promise that you will be open and honest with those who are trying to help you and that you will follow their instructions not once, but for a whole year.
4. Then determine that every time suicide enters your mind you will call a hotline *immediately.*
5. Throw out any object that makes you think of suicide. Drop friends and activities that depress you. Make new friends and find new activities.
6. Finally, if your home situation is making you suicidal, call a government office that deals with family problems, a women's shelter, a PREGNANCY AIDgency, a member of the clergy, or a hotline and tell the person who answers the phone about your situation. You may be able to live in a foster home, a group home, or government housing, or with a friend or relative. You need a supportive, positive environment where you can learn to feel good about yourself and discover and use your abilities.

You can feel different about life in a year. Then give yourself another year of life. You will still have crises to face, emotional wounds to heal, and skills to learn. With counseling, the road ahead will be a lot smoother than the road you're on.

Sixteen-year-old Maggie made her third suicide attempt when her drug-addicted boyfriend got her pregnant. Placed in a mental institution for the third time, she, with her counselor's support, was planning an abortion when her father asked a member of the clergy and a PREGNANCY AIDgency volunteer to speak to her. Maggie resented their visit, but began to rethink her decision when the AIDgency volunteer sent her an encouraging note. Maggie called the PREG-

NANCY AIDgency, which sent her to a home for unwed mothers, and then to live with a foster family. Enduring her rebellion, the foster family, through their example, led Maggie back to the faith she had rejected for seven years.

Maggie made an adoption plan. Two years later she married, and is now the happy mother of three additional children. She feels that giving birth to her baby, despite her own self-hatred, was the turning point of her life.

LIVING WITH DYING

Facing your death at the beginning of your baby's life is a bittersweet time. Confusion and fear mingle with anticipation and hope.

Begin to plan for the future by getting sound medical advice from compassionate and informed doctors. Know exactly what your risks and chances are. Your decisions are only as wise as the information on which you base them. Seek help from a PREGNANCY AIDgency and reach out to friends and relatives. Soon you will know which of them will support you. If you have a relationship with God, seek spiritual help from a member of the clergy and in prayer.

You have a say in your baby's future. Make plans and never stop hoping. Life has a way of working out for those who hope and trust. Your days ahead may be brighter if you work to make them so.

"Love is always ready to excuse, to trust,
to hope, and to endure whatever comes."

—1 Corinthians 13:7

Making Parenting Plans for the Special Needs or Dying Child

Hearing that your baby has special needs or is dying overwhelms you with confusion and grief. The diagnosis must be incorrect! How can this be happening? In vain, you search for a doctor, technology, or medication to cure your baby. Feeling helpless and out of control, bitter and angry, you see your baby as a human "time bomb."

If you continue the pregnancy, you'll begin to see each day as one more day of nurture. As you make realistic plans, you'll respond lovingly to your child.

Learning that a home for special needs children would care for their Down Syndrome son if they couldn't, Bess and Gene decided to continue the pregnancy even as they mourned intensely for the intelligent son they'd never have.

At three months of age, the infant began an early educational stimulation program. Ten years later, the child speaks well, reads at the first grade level, and is in a special classroom in a regular school. He enjoys bowling, arts and crafts, swimming, and camping. Although Bess admits that she's had some trying moments, she laughingly says, "He's a neat kid, and we love him for who he is. Trade him? Never!"

Darlene, whose story follows, told her doctor, "My child has special needs and is special to me." A child with special needs or health problems requires a special love. Not every family can give this love. Your decisions will forever influence your child's life and yours. Both of you must reach your potential. You may choose to parent your child or you may choose foster care, adoption, or institutional care. By answering the questions in Appendix G, you can explore every parenting option so that you make the best plan.

OBTAINING TREATMENT FOR YOUR CHILD

You began to parent your child when you decided to give birth. Ask your doctor if vitamins, medication, or surgery can help your baby before birth. Request treatment for your child, and choose a doctor who will aggressively treat an unhealthy child regardless of whether the child has special needs. Darlene feels that her doctor did not properly treat her son.

> *Thirty-seven-year-old Darlene had three living children and six miscarriages. When prenatal tests confirmed that her unborn son had Down Syndrome, her doctor, Dr. Smith, wanted Darlene to abort, and sent her and her husband to a genetic counselor who told them what the worst possible outcome could be. Even the ultrasound technician, who said that the baby's heartbeat was strong, told Darlene, "You won't have an abortion no matter what I say, will you?" Darlene had to tell everyone that her baby "deserves a chance, like everyone else."*
>
> *When Darlene was six months pregnant, she was in a car accident and began spotty bleeding that continued throughout the pregnancy. Dr. Smith told her that the placenta, not the baby, was probably injured. If the baby were injured, doctors could do nothing.*
>
> *At Darlene's eight-and-a-half-month checkup, the baby's heartbeat had dropped, but Dr. Smith said it was "within normal limits." About an hour after Darlene took a three-hour glucose tolerance test, the baby went into a frenzy of movement and then was still. Five days later, Darlene demanded an ultrasound which confirmed that the baby had died. Grief stricken, Darlene asked that the doctors induce labor, then do an autopsy, which found nothing unusual about the baby other than Down Syndrome.*
>
> *Dr. Jones later told Darlene that Dr. Smith must have known that her baby was in trouble when the heartbeat dropped. Had the baby been normal, Dr. Smith likely would have done an emergency Cesarean section, but he had decided that saving a Down Syndrome child's life was not worth the risk of Cesarean section to overweight Darlene. If the couple had known that their baby was in trouble, they could have found another doctor or insisted that the Cesarean be done.*

When Darlene became pregnant again, she sought a different doctor who would treat a special needs child more aggressively than Dr. Smith had. Asking a doctor the questions on medical difficulties in Appendices E and G can help you choose a doctor, too.

If a medical crisis arises or if your doctor seems to make light of a health problem (as Dr. Smith did), ask your doctor about treatment options. If your doctor says it would be hopeless to treat your child, be sure that the prognosis is accurate. Your doctor may be uninformed, may think that your child is "better off dead," or may want to spare you the emotional strain and financial burden of caring for your child.

Obtain a second and third opinion—quickly, if necessary—by calling other doctors and detailing the problem *without* mentioning that your child also has special needs or a terminal illness. Also call national groups that work with people who have children with the same special needs or illness as your child. These groups can suggest ways to deal with your child's disability or illness and may advise you of the different treatments and therapies available and of your child's prognosis.

If most children with that medical difficulty would receive treatment, but your doctor doesn't recommend it, you must decide if you want treatment and who will administer it.

Certainly any treatment that is life saving or life enhancing should be performed regardless of whether it is done prenatally or after birth. Any treatment that would unquestionably be administered to a "normal" child should probably be given. If death is imminent, that is, if your child will die within hours regardless of anything you can do, you'll probably want to refuse treatments that would merely delay your child's death.

FIRST PHYSICAL CONTACT

The more handling and touching a child experiences, the more that child will develop physically and mentally. Beginning in the hospital, hold and touch your baby frequently. Have relatives or friends spend time with the baby. An elderly person or a nursing home resident may enjoy holding the baby, too. If others will be parenting your baby, they should make contact. Or ask a doctor, hospital, church, or PREGNANCY AIDgency to help you locate parenting substitutes for your baby.

If your child returns to the hospital, see that she or he receives extensive touching and loving. Hang mobiles above your child's bed or tape colorful pictures next to it. Also bring toys to the hospital to amuse your child. This will help your child heal faster, feel secure, and develop mentally.

When their newborn needed several operations, Dwayne and Orlena spent days in the hospital, touching him, playing music, and speaking and singing to him. Because music had such a soothing effect, they began a career writing spiritual children's songs. Their son has grown into a healthy teen.

LONG-TERM PARENTING

You'll probably consider parenting your child yourself. Speak to families, foster families, and institutions that are parenting children with special needs or terminal illnesses, or consult local, state, and national agencies that deal with these children. Also join a support group for families of special needs or dying children. Visit some of these families and observe their parenting techniques. Ask as many questions as you like. Learn what help is available and decide if you can parent. Divorced with twins, both of whom had severe disabilities, and another child, Ella helped organize a support group for families with special needs children. The parents help each other and lobby for better services for their children.

Find out exactly how much medical treatment and equipment will cost and if insurance or government medical aid will pay for it. An accountant or insurance agent can help with financial planning. A university engineering department may be able to design custom equipment for your child. Surgery may correct any unusual physical appearances or life-affecting deformities. If you can't pay, make your plight public. Speak to a doctor, hospital, religious group, or PREGNANCY AIDgency. Contact a newspaper; the press may be interested in your story. Community or church groups may raise money to help you, and individual donors may make grants.

When Nellie's twins were born during her twenty-third week of pregnancy, only one survived. This child required expensive equipment to monitor his breathing, and amassed huge medical bills. Nellie had to quit her job to care for her son, and Otto's jobs couldn't pay all their expenses. The couple was ineligible for public assistance.

Following a newspaper feature on their dilemma, Nellie and Otto received donations of food, money, a better car, medical help, an expenses-paid night out, and clothing, as well as ongoing financial aid. An agency hired Nellie to do at-home mailing. A year later, a follow-up article brought additional help.

Education

Intense exercises and games help special needs children develop to full potential. A support group, pediatrician, or hospital may refer you to an early intervention program. Certain books can help you organize such a program for your child.

Many children with special needs or health problems are taught in public schools in special classes, vocational classes, or regular classrooms. Your child can function, as much as possible, as a self-supporting citizen. Arrange for home tutoring or other instruction if your child's health problems interfere with regular school attendance.

Often school or government programs provide educational opportunities and financing. You may have to inquire about these programs, or your child may have to take certain tests before being admitted. Sign your consent for testing only when you fully understand the tests, their classification systems, and what programs they apply to. With parents of other children who have special needs or health problems, fight for your child's educational rights.

Donna's newborn was paralyzed from the neck down. Donna sent him to a children's hospital, where he received physical and speech therapy along with the usual grade school subjects. After learning to use a headpointer to type, he excelled in computer science in high school classes for those with activity limita-

tions. After graduation, he worked in the computer in
own business in computers and electronic aids for persc

Parenting Help

If you need help, look for live-in, part-time, or babys
Sometimes government funds can pay for this help
for expanded services. Make a list of the kinds of help yo
friends who say, "If you need my help, just ask." You might
volunteer to grocery shop, go to the library, babysit for two hours, or
over to play with your child.

You're going to get a lot of parenting advice from friends, relatives, and professionals. Weigh what you hear and use this book to back up any plans you make. Only you know which parenting plan is best for you.

> Doctors advised Michelle and her husband to institutionalize their daughter, who was born with cerebral palsy, since she would never speak, hear, or function normally. Instead, they parented and educated the child, even giving her music lessons. When the young woman was a junior in college, over 60 percent of her body was severely burned in a fire. She survived because her mother insisted that doctors administer treatment.
>
> Today Michelle's daughter cannot dress or use the toilet herself, or write. But she is a professional counselor in private practice who writes by dictating to a secretary, and lectures widely on the problems of people with disabilities. A personal nurse helps care for her. She is determined to have others treat persons with disabilities with respect.

As your child grows, you may notice traits that doctors or social workers could miss. Call these to the attention of the professionals. Your child may exceed expectations. Doctors thought that Christopher Nolan, severely brain damaged due to a traumatic birth, was a hopeless case. His mother, however, detected signs of intelligence and had Christopher educated. He is an accomplished poet today.

Your partner and your other children need your attention, too. Take the time to do special things with them—and remember to take time out each week just for yourself. Everyone in your family needs love and nurturing, including you.

THE TERMINALLY ILL CHILD

What if a fatal condition will eventually cause your child to die? You will have to parent your child through medical crises and the stages of death. Terminally ill people receive many treatments that improve and extend their lives but do not cure their illnesses. The previous section as well as this one will help you decide if you can parent a child with a fatal condition.

Your child may live a short while or many years before dying. Tay-Sachs victims gradually lose both their physical and mental abilities and usually die before the age of four. Victims of cystic fibrosis have difficulty breathing, because of abnormally thick body mucus, and live into their teens and beyond. So do victims of muscular dystrophy, a disease of progressive muscle degeneration. Children with Wilson's

causes an abnormal accumulation of copper in the body, will have
for eight to twenty years and can be treated with drugs. Victims of
n's chorea, a progressive disease of the nervous system, live normal lives
disease begins in midlife.

ional research groups and hospitals know the latest drugs and treatments to
ng and improve life for children with terminal illnesses. While these groups
give you the latest prognosis for your child, remember that a new treatment or
ure may be around the corner. Face the future with hope as well as realism.

Parenting a dying child means overcoming the anticipation of death and living
in the present. Don't deny your baby your love to protect yourself from grief.
Know what you are facing by talking to your doctor, a national group (Appendix
H), a counselor to the dying, and other parents of terminally ill children. Visit
some children with terminal illnesses. Are you emotionally and physically strong
enough to parent your child?

A hospice can help your family and your child through the final stages of death.
If a hospital cannot refer you to a hospice in your area, a PREGNANCY
AIDgency, religious group, or civic group may be able to find volunteers to help
you a day or two a month. A counselor or member of the clergy can help you confront your emotions and live one day at a time. Those who care for your child will
grow in their ability to love, to give of themselves, and to hope in the face of despair.

ALTERNATE PARENTING PLANS

Making an alternate parenting plan requires courage and honesty. You're making
the best choice for both you and your baby. Don't feel guilty about it.

Many excellent group homes exist for special needs and terminally ill children.
Appendix H lists a few of them. A hospital, church, doctor, or PREGNANCY
AIDgency may be able to refer you to a home in your area. If one home cannot
take your child, ask for a referral to another home. When you find a home that
seems promising, visit it. Observe how the employees care for the children. Speak
to the personnel. Discuss financial arrangements. What expenses are your responsibility? What are covered by insurance, the government, private grants, or the
home? In the best homes, children receive loving care.

Tammy and Mitzie both chose institutional care for their children.
For a while, Tammy and Harold parented their daughter Joy, who had multi-
ple disabilities. Then they placed her in an institution until their other children
were older and family finances were more stable. The whole family visited Joy fre-
quently until they brought her home again.
Calvin, one of Mitzie and Lane's newborn twins, required constant care. His
parents selected an institution to become his legal guardian. Visiting often, they
were pleased at the loving treatment he received until his death.

Adoption is a choice for your special needs or terminally ill child, too. When
Dora and Oscar discovered that their unborn baby was mentally retarded, they

made an adoption plan and tried again for a normal, healthy baby. As Dora and Oscar discovered, many families are eager to adopt special needs or ill children. Perhaps you already know such a family. You can also contact a local, state, or national adoption agency, service, or lawyer. Call national agencies that work on behalf of children with special needs or terminal illnesses (see Appendix H). Their personnel may be able to put you in touch with some adoption agencies. If your child is adopted, you may be able to keep in touch with the adoptive family and visit your child. Yetta and Zack have adopted seven children with severe multiple disabilities and Dave and Neala have adopted three. These disabilities include profound retardation, physical limitation, and terminal illness. The couples call these children "rays of sunshine, God's blessings, special gifts of love." Some of the children have parents who keep in touch with the adoptive families.

Foster care, usually located through adoption or child welfare agencies, can be a good option if your child has only a short time to live. Salina has cared for nearly forty foster children over a fifteen-year period, many of them with multiple disabilities, some dying, others with brain damage so severe that they had only the most minimal brain function. The government may pay for foster care. Visit your child and the foster family so you'll feel good about your choice.

If you decide to parent your child, but then change your mind, you can make another plan at any time. Rita and Quinn brought home their child, who had severe disabilities and was dying, but found that they simply could not care for this newborn. As they arranged to place her in county-financed foster care, the infant died.

An adoption agency, member of the clergy, counselor, or PREGNANCY AIDgency can help you work through the many emotions you will experience when you consider alternate parenting plans. If your child is dying, a hospice or member of the clergy will help you deal with grief.

ACCEPTANCE

Having a child with special needs or severe health problems changes your life. You must resolve your feelings of anger, despair, and confusion, accept reality, and plan for the future. Desire your child to be all that she or he can be, not all that you wish your child were. "I am who I am, and that's all that I ever can be." A brilliant child may change the world; a child with special needs or health problems may change you.

By making a parenting plan, you acknowledge your child's worth and dignity as well as your own. Both of you deserve an environment in which you can thrive. The challenge, a nurse told a World Federation of Doctors, is to interact with the special needs child on the levels that the child can share—touch, recognition, gentleness, stimulation, presence, and love. Your parenting plan will share these qualities with your child. Your special needs or ill child will never give the world all that a well child could. Depending on your attitude, your child could give much more.

*"If I knew then
What I know now,*

You never would have died.
I'd have held you close
And nurtured you, and kept you
by my side.
I'd have sung you songs
And treasured you
More than silver,
More than gold;
But this song is all I'll give
To the babe I'll never hold."

—An anonymous woman who experienced an abortion

Dealing With Previous Abortion

You may have had an abortion in the past. An abortion procedure involves violence. Your baby died violently. You may have aborted amid violent emotional upheaval in your life. Now you may understand that you could have given birth. The knowledge that you can never reclaim your baby can torment you. You may hide your painful memories through addictions, sexual excess, wild or deviant behavior, or extreme commitment to career. Now pregnant, you may be remorseful over an abortion.

Why did you abort the last time? Family, friends, your partner, or a clinic counselor may have thought abortion was best for you. You may have felt guilty or upset over your pregnancy and chose to end it without outside pressure from anyone. You probably didn't hate your baby; you just wanted to simplify your life, and abortion seemed like the simplest solution. For a while you were glad you had the abortion, but now you may be very troubled by it. You may even wonder if you have a right to cry since you chose the procedure on your own.

Having this baby will help you understand that you do have a right to grieve. You are no longer denying your pregnancy or your baby—you are admitting to yourself that your baby is dead and that you have forever lost all contact with your child. PREGNANCY AIDgency volunteers and those who specialize in post-abortion counseling, as well as other women who regret their abortions, will help you work through your feelings.

You will have to confront your memories, your regrets, and your reasons for getting an abortion, then forgive others, your baby, and yourself for the role each played in your choice. Letting go of painful memories takes time. You may want to name your aborted baby or have a special memorial service for your child. Eventually, you may consider helping other women who are uncertain about getting abortions.

If your body suffered damage during the abortion, you may need medical treatment. If your injuries were extensive and/or permanent, a lawyer can advise you about suing an abortion clinic or abortionist for what happened to you physically during your "safe," legal abortion.

Do you need help in having this baby or making parenting choices and arrangements? A counselor can help you understand why you don't have to abort again. Regretting previous abortions, Valerie (Chapter Two), Jayne (Chapter Six), and Mercedes (Chapter Eight) went on to give birth. Bonnie, who also had a previous abortion, was working to put herself through college when she became pregnant following a vicious rape that left her almost dead. Bonnie continued her education and her job and is now parenting her baby. You, too, can lay the past to rest and build a future for yourself and your child.

". . . such a tiny thing,
A bud that had not opened,
A song too pure to sing."

—*Alice Briley*

Living Even Though Your Baby Is Dying

One in four women experience the death of their unborn or newly born babies. Often death comes unexpectedly. Other times prenatal tests indicate that the unborn child is dying. If you have had a test, request a second test to confirm the diagnosis of a fatal condition. In rare cases, prenatal tests give false positive results. You can never be 100 percent certain that your baby will die until death actually occurs. Appendix E has questions to ask in this situation.

Ectopic pregnancy, discussed earlier in this chapter, will almost always result in your child's death.

Miscarriage (spontaneous abortion) is the spontaneous ending of a pregnancy before the twentieth week and is signaled by bleeding from the vagina. Miscarriage may occur for any number of reasons.

A **stillbirth** occurs when a baby is born dead after the twentieth week of pregnancy. Babies who die in the womb suffer **intrauterine death**. If the baby is born alive, but before term, the baby is **premature**.

If a pregnancy continues several weeks beyond the anticipated due date, the baby is termed **postmature**. Postmaturity can be dangerous to the child because the placenta may cease to work well when it is too old.

A **genetic condition** has been with the child since conception; the condition is in the child's genes. Some genetic conditions are fatal while others are not.

A **congenital condition** happened to the child after conception, either due to influences in the womb or during birth. Some congenital conditions are fatal.

Infant death brings many, many questions. Discuss with your doctor how you can prevent future pregnancy loss.

TESTS

A simple pregnancy test may not tell you if your baby has died. Pregnancy tests are very sensitive to even a tiny amount of pregnancy hormones in your urine or bloodstream. The level of pregnancy hormones climbs daily as your baby grows.

When your baby dies, the hormonal level drops each day. However, enough hormones may be present to give a positive pregnancy test. This is what happened to Lynn, Gisele, and Clarissa, whose stories appear in this chapter. They had pregnancy tests register positive days after their babies had probably died.

Ask your doctor for a pregnancy test that measures your *hormonal level*. Take the test over in a few days and see if the level is rising or falling. Is the level near the normal limit and rising? Your baby is probably all right. Bed rest, hormonal treatment, or some other technique may avert disaster. Is the level very far below normal and falling? Your baby has probably died. Take the test one more time, a few days later, to be sure.

Advanced ultrasound procedures are proving that many more pregnancies than previously thought begin as twins. Bleeding early in pregnancy may indicate the death of one twin but not the other. If your hormonal levels drop, and then begin to rise again in a few days, you were pregnant with twins. One has died but the other is alive. The living twin may be fine, as Abby's twin was (Chapter Four), or may also die, as happened to Trudy (Chapter Four) during one of her miscarriages.

Many times, pregnancy loss resolves itself. You may miscarry or give birth to a dead child. Bleeding will continue for days, weeks, and possibly over a month, but will end by itself. Sometimes, bleeding is prolonged or very profuse. A doctor may think that some matter is lodged in your womb and may suggest a minor surgical procedure to be sure that your womb is empty and can heal without danger of infection.

Before consenting to any surgical procedure, have a hormonal level pregnancy test and possibly ultrasound to be sure that you are not carrying a living baby.

Many women state that the sounds and sights that occur during certain surgical procedures are upsetting. They prefer to be asleep. Other women opt for being awake, and possibly even refuse painkillers, so that they will physically confront their child's death. Although your doctor may not ask you what you prefer to do, state whether you wish to be put to sleep for any procedure. Your choice may differ from the doctor's usual routine.

BEATING THE ODDS

If death has not already occurred, you may be able to help your baby live. Some pioneers in prenatal infant psychology advise telling your baby of your love and your dreams. Your child may sense your concern. Ask your doctor if surgery, medication, vitamins, hormonal treatments, environmental changes, or bed rest may save your child. Since one doctor may be willing to try a technique that another doctor may overlook, get a second and third opinion.

> *Despite their doctors' dire predictions about their babies' ability to survive, Leslie and Roberta both did all they could to help their children live.*
>
> *Doctors advised Leslie to abort her dying unborn baby because his stomach had not closed and his bowels were outside his body. Instead Leslie continued the pregnancy. The baby underwent surgery immediately after he was born and is doing well today.*

Roberta had several miscarriages and had to remain in bed for four months to prevent another one. During one pregnancy, her water broke when she was five months pregnant. Although doctors told her that the baby could not possibly survive and was probably "defective," Roberta went on complete bed rest and gave birth two months early. Her premature son is fine today. During another pregnancy, Roberta had to stay in bed for months because she developed placenta previa, a condition in which the placenta develops too low in the womb, where it may detach early in pregnancy and endanger the baby. The child was born full term. During each of these crises, friends from church and prayer groups brought meals and did housecleaning. Roberta's husband and other children helped, too.

Be aware of your unborn baby's movements. Report any underactivity or overactivity to your doctor. Your baby's radically changed behavior pattern may be your first indication that something is wrong. A quick delivery may save your baby's life. When doctors could not detect any vital signs on two monitoring machines, they declared Ami Zilembo, twenty-seven days overdue, as stillborn. After a quick Cesarean section, Ami was born alive and is a healthy child today.

Request tests if you are two weeks or more past your due date. Your baby's placenta may be functioning less efficiently, and delivery might be wise.

Prematurity

If premature labor threatens, let your doctor know that you are determined to carry your baby as long as possible. Check with a large city hospital on the latest techniques, treatments, and technologies to prevent premature labor. Ask your doctor to try these. Follow your doctor's instructions, try to remain calm, and count each day as a victory. This is what Abby and Barb (Chapter Four) and Roberta (this chapter) did. They were able to stop premature labor, at least for a time.

Very small premature infants sometimes survive. Trent Petrie, born twenty-two weeks after conception and weighing only twelve ounces, survived because his parents chose life support systems for him. Today, although functionally blind due to his extreme prematurity, Trent is otherwise healthy.

Jacqueline Benson also weighed twelve ounces at birth and survived. Four months premature, Monica Mere weighed thirteen ounces and was delivered early because her mother was suffering from a disease in which the liver fails and the blood system stops its clotting process. Both Monica and her mother are healthy today.

Babies born six months after conception have over a **50** percent chance of survival. Most will have few, if any, permanent difficulties. Breast milk is the best food for preemies. If your child is too small to nurse, pump your breasts and give your baby breast milk by bottle or feeding tube. Breastfeeding support groups can advise on breastfeeding premature infants. Despite your child's tubes, wires, monitors, and machines, determine to speak to, touch, and play with your baby as much as possible, as did Kelsey and Vance, whose daughter was born three-and-a-half months early. Their incredibly long hours at the hospital resulted in a daughter who is now developing normally. Their child, like all premature babies, thrived on human attention and stimulation.

LOVING THE UNBORN BABY WHO HAS NO CHANCE OF SURVIVAL

The knowledge that your baby is dying within you can evoke the most brutal emotions you will ever face. Your decision to allow your baby's birth and death to take place naturally may meet great opposition. However, many mothers who know that their babies can't survive still choose to give birth.

Monica was seven months pregnant when ultrasound revealed that her unborn baby had no kidneys and would be unable to survive outside her womb. The baby was becoming less and less active as his own body wastes poisoned his system. Monica's doctor began to monitor the pregnancy weekly. If the baby died and Monica did not go into labor, the doctor could induce labor to prevent the baby from infecting Monica if his body began to decompose.

Monica cherished each day that her baby lived, and imagined that he was warm and comfortably relaxed in her womb. When Monica went into labor a month early, she and her husband had the baby baptized. After doctors confirmed the child's condition, Monica and her husband had the life-support system disconnected from their baby and held him until he died in their arms. Monica treasures her memories of that morning with her son.

If doctors determine that your baby will be unable to survive after birth, some people may try to persuade you to end your pregnancy early. Even though you may want to carry your baby to term, others may argue against this decision. Following are some suggested responses to comments or questions that you may hear.

"Why continue the pregnancy when your baby has no chance of survival?"
"I know that my doctor probably is correct with the diagnosis, but I want to make absolutely sure by having my baby tested after birth. If the prenatal test results are wrong, I want my baby treated."

"You won't be getting an abortion. You'll just be ending your pregnancy early."
"My baby is still alive. Even a healthy baby couldn't survive being born this prematurely."

"You'll lose valuable time in conceiving a healthy baby if you don't end this pregnancy."
"My cervical and uterine muscles aren't ready to deliver my baby yet. If labor is induced or if I get an abortion now, those muscles might be weakened. I don't want to take that chance because it might cause me to miscarry or to deliver my next baby prematurely."

"You are only a life-support system for your dying baby. Why don't you disconnect the life support?"

"Every pregnant woman is *naturally* a life-support system for her unborn baby. When my baby is born, I won't choose *artificial* life support."

"Your unborn baby is suffering."
"Babies who die after birth often die peacefully. My baby may not be suffering at all. If I thought that my baby was in pain, I would ask my doctor to do something to ease the pain."

"Your baby might die and start to decompose inside you. Geneticists can't use decayed cells to determine what caused your baby's problems or whether they can happen again."
"If I were concerned about this, I'd request an amniocentesis before my baby dies. Geneticists can examine my baby's cells to determine if the problems are genetic in origin. In addition, my doctor is checking me weekly. If my baby dies and I don't go into labor, I'll have labor induced so that my baby won't start to decompose." (Refer to Chapter Four for a discussion of amniocentesis.)

"It would be better for you emotionally to end this pregnancy now."
"I don't think so. I'll admit that sometimes I do feel hopeless, angry, and unable to endure one more day. But that's how most people feel at times if they're caring for a terminally ill loved one. By allowing my pregnancy to end naturally, I won't ever wonder if my baby might have lived. I'm in touch with people who are helping me deal with my grief [perhaps a hospice or a support group for parents who experienced infant loss]. I am cherishing each day that my baby lives even though I am making funeral plans."

When your baby is born, you will probably be amazed by your child's beauty despite any abnormal features. If your baby dies, you will gradually get on with your life, but you will never forget your baby. Time does not erase that kind of love.

> When Marcia learned that her thirty-two-week-old unborn daughter was deformed and dying, she wanted the pregnancy over, now. Her doctor refused to induce labor. Marcia's hatred, anger, and bitterness toward her baby slowly evolved into love. Even as she made funeral arrangements, she prayed that her baby would live a while. The dying newborn had abnormal features but was still beautiful. Asking that the child be taken off a respirator, Marcia and her husband held and caressed the baby as she died slowly and peacefully. Family members grieved a long time, but are glad that they had a natural birth experience.

PARENTING THE DYING NEWBORN

"I didn't forget to run my fingers along
her pug nose and talk to her in my lingo . . .
"I didn't forget to take pictures of her
and note the color of her eyes.

> *"I didn't forget to cry in front of her*
> *and beg her to get better . . ."*

—*Marion Cohen,* Intensive Care #2

If your child is born alive but dying, you will face life's most bittersweet experience—nurturing an infant while watching life ebb away. Love and comfort your child while death comes, as did Monica and Marcia, whose stories appear earlier in this chapter.

If your child is suffering, speak to a doctor about it. Almost always, drugs and technologies can greatly reduce or eliminate suffering. Loving and touching can also help your child feel much better.

DEATH OF A TWIN

If you are pregnant with more than one child, one or more of your babies may die, leaving other children alive. This happened to Abby (Chapter Four). The need to both grieve and rejoice, to release and to bond, can be confusing. Fearing the death of your living children, you may become overprotective of them.

Speak about your dead babies. Find out why they died. Have a baptism or dedication service for your living children, a memorial service for your dead ones. Grieve at times and rejoice at others.

Children seem to retain a subconscious sense of togetherness with dead siblings, probably because they were womb mates. This manifests itself in drawings and conversation, even if the living children were not told of the dead ones.

When your children are old enough, tell a story about the ill siblings who died and how sad you felt. Tell your living children how happy you are that they are alive. Assure them that they did nothing to cause the death. This story will pave the way for additional questions later. Answer questions openly. Accept emotions as they arise.

> *When Sue spontaneously aborted one twin, she had to separate rage from hope. Ill throughout the pregnancy, she struggled through postpartum depression to bond with the living twin. She feels that the baby senses the loss of his brother, and she plans to tell him about his sibling when he is older.*

SAYING GOOD-BYE

You will have your own way of saying good-bye. You may choose never to see your baby, or you may try one or more of the suggestions listed below. Talk over what you can emotionally handle with someone you trust or a member of a hospital staff or national support group for parents experiencing infant death (see Appendix H).

You may wish to hold your baby. Tenderly wrap the baby (or the remains) in a soft cloth or blanket. Holding your baby makes your child's life and death real and affirms your right to grieve. If your child is alive, you will be able to caress your infant as death, which is often peaceful, comes. You may wish to photograph your baby.

After many fertility treatments, René became pregnant. When the baby stopped moving eight weeks before his due date, doctors performed an emergency Cesarean section and discovered that the baby had no brain activity. In consultation with doctors, Ed and René had the baby removed from a respirator. They held, caressed, photographed, and videotaped their five-day-old son, who died in their arms. René's bitter feelings toward women with healthy babies took a while to resolve. Having mementos of the birth helped. So did an autopsy report that helped René realize that she could not have prevented the death. The baby had a genetic brain abnormality which caused his death.

Before any surgical procedure begins, tell your doctor if you'd like to hold your baby's remains or have them for a funeral. Many doctors never consider that a woman would want the remains. If a lab must perform tests on the body, you can usually have the body later, if you ask.

Naming your baby acknowledges your child's existence. If you do not know your baby's sex, you may want to guess at it, or choose a unisex name such as Leslie, Sydney, Terry, Marty, Lee, Pat, Robin, or Jody.

Memorial Services

Some parents use a funeral or memorial service to say good-bye and to let others know that they are grieving. A PREGNANCY AIDgency, member of the clergy, or funeral director can help you plan. The service may be simple or elaborate, private or public, quiet or vibrant with music. You may choose cremation or burial for a baby whose body you have. Often a cemetery will bury a miscarried or stillborn baby without charge.

A funeral home may have caskets and burial vaults available for infants, small children, and miscarried babies. The smallest sizes are available through the Pregnancy and Infant Loss Center (see Appendix H).

If you anticipate that your baby may die, you may ask a funeral home to order a small casket. Hopefully, you will not need it, and the funeral home can have it on hand for someone else whose baby has died. Often funeral parlors will make free arrangements for the burial of very small infants.

You may find much comfort in holding, washing, and dressing your child for burial. Small burial gowns are available, or you can purchase an appropriate piece of newborn or doll's clothing and dress your infant. If you miscarried early in pregnancy, you can hold a memorial service regardless of whether you have the remains.

Five women memorialized the losses of their children in five touching ways.

When Gisele's first pregnancy ended in miscarriage, she wrote a poem to her baby, whom she named Grace. She and her husband memorialized Grace by taking a long walk near the ocean. Here they prayed for Grace and for themselves.

Clarissa named her three miscarried babies "Chris" and baptized each of their remains, then buried them with her family present. When she retrieved a tiny, intact five-week embryo from the third miscarriage, a member of the clergy held a private memorial service for the family. Then Clarissa and her family took the baby to the cemetery to be buried, without charge, in the stillborn vault.

When forty-three-year-old Lara's unborn baby died after Lara was beaten by her boyfriend, a PREGNANCY AIDgency that had arranged shelter for Lara now found a funeral director to donate the costs of her infant's funeral.

Betsy and Glenn planned a large funeral for their premature first child. They both readied their child for burial and participated in church readings.

After Carol and her boyfriend Wes changed their minds about having an abortion, their baby was stillborn on Christmas Day. A PREGNANCY AIDgency volunteer helped them through the grief and shock. Carol, Wes, and their parents visit the baby's grave often, bringing flowers.

If you were making an adoption plan for your baby, the adoptive family should see and handle the body and participate in any funeral arrangements or memorial services. In the book *Daddy, I'm Pregnant*, the anonymous author Bill tells how his daughter Angela and the adoptive family she had chosen both made funeral arrangements when Angela's infant daughter died.

GRIEVING

Being left childless brings a startling grief. You grieve not only for your lost motherhood, but also for the infant, toddler, child, teen, adult, and grandparent the world will never know. This will happen whether or not you intended to be pregnant.

The persistence and depth of your grief may surprise you. You have a right and a need to grieve, to be angry. Let your tears flow. Allow yourself time to feel better. You may grieve for a year or more.

Nevertheless, some people will assume that you should quickly get on with your life and conceive again. If you have one living child of a multiple birth, some individuals may wonder why you are grieving at all. And, if your pregnancy was a crisis, some people may feel that your baby's death should bring relief. In trying to encourage you, people sometimes make hurtful, insensitive remarks. Say, "Thank you for trying to encourage me. I know I'll feel better in time." Then seek out those who can understand your pain.

Talk to a relative, lover, confidant, or member of the clergy, or to another mother who experienced infant death. Call your doctor, hospital, or PREGNANCY AIDgency for referral to a support group of people who have experienced infant or child loss or who are parenting very ill or dying children. Attend meetings of this group or speak to a member by phone or in person. You will feel much love and understanding and will learn some practical ways of dealing with the future.

Darlene (earlier in this chapter) attends a support group for parents who have experienced pregnancy and infant loss. So does Amanda, whose newborn died on Christmas Eve. The meetings help Amanda to deal with her grief and anger. They are also a means of preserving her child's memory and helping other parents.

AUTOPSY

If you want to know what caused your baby's death, request an autopsy, as Ed and René did (earlier in this chapter). Ask how long it will take to get the results. Request a copy of the autopsy and have a doctor thoroughly explain it. If your doctor doesn't understand the terminology, ask other doctors or medical experts to explain the report. A PREGNANCY AIDgency may be able to find a doctor to explain the terminology to you.

If your baby had special needs or a terminal illness, doctors may wonder why you want an autopsy. However, you have a right to an autopsy no matter what your child's condition.

If you feel that someone caused your child's death—from accident, misdiagnosis, physical abuse, poor medical treatment, or another cause—a lawyer can tell you if you can sue for damages. Going to court is a costly, emotionally draining experience. If your child died before birth, it may be difficult to collect damages, as the law may not consider children to be persons until they are born. However, you may be able to collect for emotional damages.

CARE FOR THE GRIEVERS

Take care of yourself. Eat a nutritious diet and drink plenty of fluids. Avoid caffeine, which may increase tension; alcohol, a depressant; and drugs. You will heal faster if you face your emotions head on and work through them.

When your doctor allows, exercise to release tension. Rest often, even if you don't sleep. Do less. Depression may keep you from maintaining a full schedule for a while. Write down your feelings, talk about them, or tape-record them. Even if you are angry or bitter, continue your communication with God. Every so often do something you enjoy.

Maintain communication with your partner if he is still part of your life. Both of you will grieve differently. Men often conceal grief or are poor at expressing feelings. Share your feelings and open up to each other so that your relationship remains strong. Resume sexual relations when *both* of you are ready. Discuss if and when you want to conceive again. Assume nothing about your partner's feelings. Talk things over.

Help your children express their feelings about the death. Compare your baby's death to the death of someone else your children knew or to death in nature. Show your children that you love them. Let them know that nothing they thought or did caused their sister's or brother's death. Involve them in funeral or memorial services. Answer their questions honestly. Allow your children to grieve in their own unique ways and in their own time.

Some women find that helping others who are experiencing similar losses is very therapeutic. Others work with ill children. Still other women go on to parent children, either biological children or adopted children, and eventually feel whole again. One mother acknowledges the baby she miscarried in every formal portrait taken of her large family. In these portraits, one living child holds a rosebud to represent the baby who died. Even though you will always remember your baby, time truly is a great healer. Deal with your grief. Hope for the future.

> *When Isaac and Rayanne lost all five of their children to stillbirth, miscarriage, or death upon birth, they turned bitterness into love by adopting two children. Bernadette and her husband also lost five children, three to miscarriage and two to prematurity. They also have adopted two children. Bernadette is counselor of a large support group for parents grieving the loss of a child, and editor of the group's newsletter. Issac and Rayanne belong to such a group and help other hurting families.*

GIVE YOURSELF TIME

In the poem *Our Wee White Rose*, Gerald Massey wrote about the death of a child. "You scarce would think so small a thing/Could leave a loss so large." The healing process begins when you first hear that your baby is dying or dead. As you work through the anguish of death, plan a funeral or memorial service, and cry your way through the period that follows infant loss, you will begin to experience healing.

Healing takes time. Lots of it. You will get on with your life, but you will still remember losing your child. Your child will have helped you to grow, even though your child died. Memorialize your child by turning your grief into service to others.

Chapter Eight

HOPE FOR THE FUTURE

You've begun a long journey on your way to giving birth. The bleakness you saw before is becoming light. You've made selfless decisions, and you'll make more. Because of you, a child will soon be born. No one can predict how many people your child will help.

"Crisis" comes from a Greek word which means a discerning. You've faced a crisis and survived. Your crisis has helped you discern who you are and who you can be. You can never return to the you of before.

You may not be happy with the way your life has turned out to this point. Perhaps you feel that there has to be more to living than what you've experienced or felt. Maybe you want things to improve for you and your baby. You can find the peace you're looking for.

BEING A POSITIVE PERSON

You can begin to find peace by deciding to be a positive thinker. Remember the ideas in Chapter Two? They work! Build your confidence by thinking positively, by exercising to release your stress, and by doing activities that you enjoy. Know your limits. You don't have to say "yes" to every request for your time or talents. Know what you can do, and do what you can. Avoid stressful situations the way you'd avoid the flu!

Be especially aware of those who surround you. Look for optimistic friends. Avoid the negative thinkers, complainers, and depressing personalities. Their attitudes are contagious, and they'll make you depressed. Be alert to people who will use or abuse you or who constantly belittle you and your ideas. Associate with those who will increase your self-confidence, not erase it.

Usually you can find positive thinkers in community or religious groups, most often those providing service to others. When you begin to help those less fortunate than you, your own problems gain perspective. Helping others will also make you feel better about your own abilities.

Take time to be alone and to relax. Reading a good inspirational book, going on a quiet walk, or listening to soothing music may give you perspective and help you think more positively.

Remember to live one day at a time. Do your best today. Worry about tomorrow when tomorrow comes.

COUNSELING

You may have some deep emotional problems that have never been faced. These problems may have started with an abusive childhood or relationship or when peers rejected you. Perhaps you hurt yourself through substance abuse, sexual excess, self-harm, or extreme rebellion. You may not like the way you feel but not know how to change.

Counseling is a good way to get to know the root of your problems and grow through them to become a mature, happy person. Insurance companies sometimes pay for counseling performed by licensed psychologists or psychiatrists. If you have no insurance and you cannot afford to pay professionals, call a local government-sponsored mental health center. These centers often provide counseling on a sliding fee scale, which is set up according to what you can afford to pay.

Remember that some clergy are excellent professional counselors, too, and their fees are usually reasonable. A local association of clergy or churches or synagogues may be able to refer you to clergy counselors.

Be certain that the counselor you choose is in agreement with your decision to have your baby. Deal with your baby through a PREGNANCY AIDgency and use a professional counselor to help you deal with yourself.

THE TWELVE-STEP PROGRAM OF SELF-HELP GROUPS

Self-help groups generally form to help their members overcome a specific problem in their lives. Alcoholics Anonymous is probably the most widely known self-help group and follows a twelve-step program to sobriety. Many other self-help groups are based on the twelve steps of Alcoholics Anonymous. By joining one of these groups and by changing the word ''alcohol'' in step one to whatever compulsion, addiction, or worry that you are facing, you can follow the twelve-step program of Alcoholics Anonymous to a fuller, happier life.

The Twelve Steps of Alcoholics Anonymous

1. We admitted we were powerless over alcohol—that our lives had become unmanageable.
2. Came to believe that a Power greater than ourselves could restore us to sanity.
3. Made a decision to turn our will and our lives over to the care of God *as we understood Him.*
4. Made a searching and fearless moral inventory of ourselves.
5. Admitted to God, to ourselves, and to another human being the exact nature of our wrongs.

6. Were entirely ready to have God remove all these defects of character.
7. Humbly asked Him to remove our shortcomings.
8. Made a list of all persons we had harmed, and became willing to make amends to them all.
9. Made direct amends to such people wherever possible, except when to do so would injure them or others.
10. Continued to take personal inventory and when we were wrong promptly admitted it.
11. Sought through prayer and meditation to improve our conscious contact with God, *as we understood Him*, praying only for knowledge of His will for us and the power to carry that out.
12. Having had a spiritual awakening as the result of these steps, we tried to carry this message to alcoholics, and to practice these principles in all our affairs.*

Working the twelve-step program takes a lifetime. Most people take several months just to work through step one. You need an equally long time to work up to and achieve the other steps. Overcoming a lifetime problem will take a lifetime, so be patient. The twelve-step program is obviously successful. So many people are using it every day, and just starting on the program will bring some positive changes to your life.

You do not have to be battling the specific problem of a self-help group in order to be helped by it. Attend meetings of different self-help groups. Find one that follows the twelve-step program and whose members make you feel comfortable being there. If you can't find a self-help group, consider starting your own.

If you find a self-help group that follows a program other than the twelve-step program, evaluate what you hear and observe. Does the program seem to work? Do the members seek to change their unhealthy ways of coping with life in general, or are they simply present to support each other in dealing with a specific crisis, such as suicide of a loved one or death of a child? Decide if the group can help you, and stay if it does.

Agencies in Appendix H will help you locate or start self-help groups in your area.

God in the Twelve-Step Program

You'll notice that the twelve-step program is based on a belief in the power of God as you understand God to be. Twelve-step programs do not advocate a certain religious view. Whether God is male or female or whether one religion is "right" in its beliefs is not the point. Ninety-four percent of United States citizens believe in God or a universal spirit, according to the Princeton Religion Research Center Gallup Poll. You will find many believers and seekers in self-help groups.

---

*The Twelve Steps are reprinted with permission of Alcoholics Anonymous World Services, Inc. Permission to reprint the steps does not mean that AA has reviewed or approved the contents of this publication nor that AA agrees with the views expressed herein. AA is a program of recovery from alcoholism. Use of these Twelve Steps in connection with programs and activities which are patterned after AA, but which address other problems, does not imply otherwise.

Sponsors

Most self-help groups based on the twelve-step program will provide you with a sponsor, if you request one. A sponsor is a member of the group who has followed the twelve-step program for a reasonable period of time and, by doing so, has successfully managed the problem addressed by the group. This person will guide you in your own journey and become a great friend and adviser. If you want a sponsor when you join a self-help group, go to many meetings before choosing one. Get to know the group members. Choose a sponsor who seems to be practicing the twelve steps successfully and who has the inner peace you are seeking for yourself.

RELIGIOUS PRAYER GROUPS

Many churches, synagogues, and other religious groups can direct you to prayer groups or other religious support groups. The members of these groups most often have a certain religious orientation. If you practice a specific faith, seek out a prayer group of that faith. If you are searching for a faith experience, call local clergy and ask about prayer groups and worship services. Find a group whose members seem kind and helpful and are practicing their beliefs peacefully and joyfully.

Prayer groups can be a tremendous help in crisis. Most of the women who best survive pregnancy crisis have faith in God. Probably 90 percent of counselors in PREGNANCY AIDgencies believe in and try to trust God. A prayer group can help you develop your own faith and work through your crisis while other people support your efforts.

Prayer groups will help you develop a conscious awareness of God through prayer and meditation. You might be encouraged to read the Bible, pray daily, or attend religious services. You'll learn that the members of the prayer group love and accept you, just the way you are. So does God. Knowing this will help you forgive yourself for any poor choices you think you've made. You'll also learn to forgive others who have harmed you. You might even have to forgive God for letting bad things happen to you.

Prayer groups and worship services will help you understand that God is a real presence that surrounds you, lives in you, and cares deeply about you. God is willing to help you, but you must accept that help. Tell God about your angers, worries, frustrations, and complaints. God knows about them anyway.

A Word of Caution

Supportive prayer groups will help you deal successfully with your life, but those associated with cults will create more problems for you. Some cults use prayer groups and Bible study get-togethers to recruit new members.

Before you join a prayer group, get some information about it. What person or religious body sponsors the group? Do the members meet for regular worship? Where? What are the beliefs of the group? What demands does it make on its members? Refer to Chapter Three for additional tips on how to determine if a group is trying to control you. Appendix F has questions to consider when evaluating a group. Also have some friends or counselors evaluate the group before you join it.

Avoid prayer groups and Bible study groups that have bizarre ideas, follow charismatic leaders, make demands on their members, are unclear about the way they originated, or persuade their members to conform to unusual dietary, dress, or behavior patterns. A supportive prayer group helps its members find God in their own diversity. A cult-run group persuades its members to conform to a lifestyle and adopt someone else's ideas. If all the loving, supportive, long-time members of a group seem to be clones of each other in their ideas and lifestyles, then you may be dealing with a cult. Call some established religious groups in your community and locate a more mainstream prayer group to help you.

HELPING OTHERS

"No one is where they are by accident," one member of the clergy said. You have a purpose in life. You will slowly come to realize what it is. Maybe no one else can do what you can do, right now, right here. Your own deepest hurts may make you more sensitive to the pain others feel. Someday you may be helping them.

You have talents and abilities you may not recognize. Not everyone can do everything well, but each of us can do some things better than other people can. For example, a child who consistently failed reading in school became a success in life by using a talent in construction to work for a contractor and the government and to build the family's home. You can use your talents to help yourself and others.

Soon you will meet people who can use your help. Some people will accept your advice and help, while others won't. What's important is that you have the inner peace and direction to help. You have changed and grown.

Although Mercedes came from a loving family, she was raised without values or direction. She ran with a fast crowd, wondered who she was, and even considered suicide. When she became pregnant, she aborted her baby, whose existence seemed as meaningless as her own. Now she felt even worse.

Mercedes' friends didn't want to talk about what was hurting her. Then she met John, who regretted helping a girlfriend get an abortion. Both uncomfortable with their friends, they shared their thoughts and hurts with each other. Together they continued a search for God that John had begun. Was there meaning to existence? Did an Objective Truth exist?

The two married and were struggling financially when Mercedes became pregnant. Delighted even though they were poor, they continued to study various faiths, then joined a religious group that they felt held the truth they sought. A member of the clergy helped both of them forgive themselves and experience God's forgiveness, too.

Since both had been hurt by shallow friends and by abortion, John and Mercedes decided to be real friends to women in pregnancy crises and help them have their babies. Soon others joined them. Today this group helps many women. John and Mercedes' closeness to God, their family, and others continues to be strong.

THE JOURNEY OF A LIFETIME

Living is a journey. The roads we choose now lead to our future. However, a lifetime is not long enough to "make it" to our destination of total peace, happiness, and trust. We are always in the process of learning more about ourselves, of dealing more wisely with others, and of trusting more deeply in God.

If you want peace and hope in your life, you must start someplace. The suggestions in this chapter will help you make a good beginning. By using self-help groups, counselors, or religious groups, and by working to think positively, you will find your life slowly gaining direction and purpose. No matter how troubled your past seems, your future can be brighter if you look ahead today. Put on a smile and get to work. All you have to gain is a lifetime of joy!

Appendix A

A SUMMARY OF PRENATAL DEVELOPMENT

The following is a summary of a baby's development in the womb.

- Within the first hours and days after conception, the baby's cells divide, taking on different forms and functions. Development is rapid and complex. The baby's heart begins beating when the mother's period is four days late.
- A good doctor, with the latest equipment, can let you hear this heartbeat when you are only six weeks pregnant. Upon doing an internal exam, the doctor can push your uterus forward against your anterior abdominal wall (tummy) and pick up your baby's heartbeat with a special ultrasonic transducer. You can record your baby's heartbeat on a cassette tape. If your doctor does not have ultrasonic equipment, you may have to wait a few weeks to hear the heartbeat.
- At two months, the baby has every organ in place, is moving vigorously, has distinctive fingerprints, and can feel pain, even though only an inch or so long.
- At three months, every baby has a unique personality and distinct features. Some babies are graceful ballerinas while others are quarterbacks, gymnasts, or soccer players. You'll soon know your baby's kicking pattern!
- A five-month-old baby has sleeping cycles. A loud noise will startle the baby. Unborn babies like soothing music and hate loud, discordant noise. A baby of this age can learn in the womb—this was proven by scientists at Prenatal University in California.
- At six months, the baby has a chance of survival if born early. Your baby is aware of your emotions and love. Your thoughts and feelings are helping the baby establish personality and security. By thinking pleasant thoughts and speaking to your baby, you build your child's confidence and help your baby feel secure and loved.
- At seven months, a baby can see light through your abdominal wall and doesn't like brightness. Reacting to extreme light, the baby will kick. A lot. Wearing a bikini to the beach may not be the best idea! Use it next summer.
- At birth, a baby will have the same sleeping, waking, and activity patterns as in the womb. Is the baby a thumb sucker? Vigorous hiccupper? Daytime sleeper—nighttime mover? The baby is continuing to act in familiar ways. Birth merely changes the location where the baby lives. Your child is a unique person from the very beginning and will remain so forever.

Appendix B

LETTER FROM AN ADULT WITH SPECIAL NEEDS

The following Letter to the Editor was printed in the Newport Daily News, *Newport, Rhode Island, on May 25, 1989. The writer has Down Syndrome, a genetic condition that causes mild to moderate mental retardation. This letter is reproduced with permission.*

The use of this letter does not imply that its author, or the organizations and individuals mentioned within the letter, adhere to any specific views regarding abortion.

To the Editor:

My name is Bob Lanouette. I have Down Syndrome. I am very smart and very bright. I was born with Down Syndrome.

This story is about Down Syndrome, and how a person with Down Syndrome learns differently. A group of people who study Down Syndrome are those belonging to an organization by the name of The National Down Syndrome Congress. They study such things as the amount of chromosomes a person has. After reading such letters from this organization I have developed many feelings about Down Syndrome.

I do not understand what causes Down Syndrome. It seems that a person is born with Down Syndrome. A Down Syndrome baby is very smart, they can walk, talk and have many learning skills but as an adult it is very hard for people to understand what it is like to have Down Syndrome.

As a Down Syndrome adult I am able to learn many new things and develop many new skills. It seems as though people do not understand that. People must learn to understand that the Down Syndrome adult has much talent and they are able to learn and grow as anybody else can learn and grow.

The Down Syndrome person can learn so much in life. They have special teachers to help them, for example, those teachers who help in the Special Olympics, or those teachers who help with speech problems. There are also those people who volunteer to help the Down Syndrome person. An example of volunteers, are those at Salve Regina College who help me develop better writing skills.

Even though a person has Down Syndrome, they are very smart. We are able to read newspapers, work on computers and like myself write poetry and stories. The Down Syndrome person has much talent and uses that talent to learn and do many new things.

Bob Lanouette
Newport, Rhode Island

Appendix C

BIRTH FOR THE MENTALLY RETARDED MOTHER

Even severely retarded women can get pregnant, either from rape or from a love relationship, and can give birth without undue fear or pain. In making decisions for the mentally retarded woman, speak to her doctor and caseworker. Medications can make pregnancy, labor, and delivery more comfortable. Help the woman understand as much as she can about pregnancy and childbirth. If she can understand, involve her in any adoption arrangements. Have the woman meet the adoptive parents and possibly visit her baby shortly after the adoption is complete. You may involve the baby's father in adoption arrangements, too.

The woman and her lover may wish to marry and parent the child. Mildly mentally retarded adults can parent well with supervision. Speak to the couple's caseworkers about the feasibility of marriage. This couple could learn parenting skills through your community mental health center. With early childhood education programs and child help groups, the couple's child can learn skills that they may have difficulty teaching.

Eudora had an IQ of seventy, and her husband Don had a learning disability. Together they raised a daughter who today teaches emotionally disturbed and mentally retarded students and who is about to enter graduate school, majoring in special education. A shy, quiet couple, Eudora and Don kept a loving, comfortable home. When neither could help their daughter with schoolwork, they told her to ask her teacher. As the girl grew older, she gradually assumed more of a parenting role to her own parents. Today she and Eudora are especially close.

Appendix D

IF YOU DON'T WANT A CHILD

You may never have wanted to have a child. If so, you have your reasons, but do you know what they are? These questions will help you discover them. Write down what is bothering you and discuss it with a counselor, confidant, or member of the clergy. Once you know why having a child seems so upsetting, you may be able to confront your emotions logically. Do your feelings reflect the truth in every situation or is your past coloring your views? Perhaps you need to talk to some parents or receive some psychological counseling. With guidance, it is possible to work through your negative emotions and give birth to your baby.

CHILDREN AND PARENTING

- Do I dislike children? Why?
- What bad experiences have I had with children?
- What have I read, heard, or observed that has formed my views?
- Do I think that I will ever change my views about children?
- What do I think of people who love children?
- Do I understand that nearly every person's view of children has some basis? What is my view of children? The view of those who love children?
- How was my relationship with my mother? Father? Why was it like that? Did I hate one or both parents?
- How am I different from either parent? Which parent do I see myself becoming if I parent a child? How do I feel about that?
- Can I change my personal parenting image?

Understand Your Childhood

- Did I know my parents?
- Was I in foster care or adopted?
- Did I grow up in a group home or facility for children?
- What attitudes do I have toward my upbringing? How do these attitudes affect me and my views of parenting?
- Was I treated badly as a child? Neglected? Abused, either physically, sexually, or emotionally?
- Did I have trouble living up to someone else's expectations? Was I never good enough?
- Did my parents treat me as if I were, or should have been, a miniature adult?
- Do I fear that I (or others) will treat my child as I was treated?
- Did I feel unwanted as a child? Unplanned? Did I seem a burden?
- Am I afraid that my child would be a burden? Be unwanted?
- Is it I or someone else who doesn't want my child?

- Am I embarrassed to admit that I don't want my baby? Do I feel guilty?
- Am I afraid that my child would hate or reject me? Would rebel? Would cause me emotional pain? Would be a financial drain?
- How do I see my unborn baby? As a glob? As a non-person? Is this how I *really* feel or am I trying to cover up or ignore my deepest knowledge that I have a child, small, not fully formed, but still a child, within me?
- Am I convincing myself that my child is a formless mass so that I can get an abortion without any regrets? Would I have any regrets? Now? Five years from now? When I'm old?

Fears of Parenting Options

- Do I feel incapable of parenting? Am I insecure?
- Why doesn't parenting fit into my view of myself?
- Would parenting interfere with my career, education, lifestyle, world view?
- Would I ever change my views about being a parent? How do I feel about that?
- Am I afraid that I will want to raise my baby if I give birth? Does that frighten me?
- What is it about motherhood that frightens or repels me? Can talking to other mothers relieve some of my fears?
- Would I want to leave my job to care for my child? Does this frighten me? Why?
- Do I know about day care or babysitting? How do I feel about these options? What about a live-in nanny, arrangements with relatives, or sharing child care with my partner?
- What are my feelings about adoption? Why do I feel this way? Can I change? Do I need more information about adoption?
- Do I think I would be foolish to go through pregnancy and then make an adoption plan? Why do I feel this way?
- Do I realize that nine months of my life can give a baby decades to live, either with me or with someone else?
- Do I know that I can keep in touch with my child if I make certain adoption plans? Is this an option for me?

MEN AND WOMEN

- What is my view of women? Of men? Do I see women as servants, men as masters? Is this just? Accurate?
- Does my value come from my sexuality? Do I feel that I must always be sexually available, always attractive?
- Do men give me a sense of worth? What is my worth without a man in my life?
- Is sex fun?
- Am I afraid this pregnancy will ruin my dating or sexual relationship? How much do I really know about sex during pregnancy? Can a doctor give me the facts?

Body Beautiful?

- How do I feel about pregnant women? What do I think pregnant women look like? How does pregnancy change my view of myself and my sex appeal?
- What is unjust in the way some men perceive pregnant women?
- Have I always feared weight gain? Do I have a thin ideal of myself? Do I think fat people are ugly? Why do I feel the way I do about my body? Is this a just viewpoint?
- Does the weight gain of pregnancy worry me more than anything else? How will pregnancy really affect my weight over a year's time?
- Can I tolerate being heavy for a brief time to give my baby a chance at a future?

- Am I afraid that pregnancy will permanently disfigure my body? Am I concerned about sagging breasts and stretch marks? Do I know that doctors can suggest exercises and creams to prevent the problems that disgust me?
- Does my lover want a perfect looking, always-available woman? Am I afraid of losing him if I am pregnant?
- Have I ever thought of how I will keep a man like this when I get old and am no longer perfect looking or always available?
- Should this man and I have a good discussion about my body and our baby? Can we agree that a less-than-perfect me might be fine for a while in order to give our baby a future?

You and Men

- Is it really my lover who never, ever wanted to have a baby? Have I been accepting his ideas without thinking for myself? How will I feel if I get an abortion because my lover wants it?
- Has physical, emotional, or sexual abuse colored my views of men and of myself?
- Is this pregnancy a result of sexual abuse?
- Do I hate men?
- Do I think that my baby is a boy and that I would hate him for being male? Why do I have these feelings? Do I want to overcome these feelings? What can I do to overcome them? Might a psychologist help?
- Do I hate myself? Have I ever thought of suicide? Do I wish I were dead sometimes? Do I wish I had never been born?
- Am I afraid that my child will have the same negative feelings that I have? How do I *know* what my child will feel?
- How can I change my feelings about myself and life? Do I want to change them?
- Do I need counseling?

Feminist Fears

- Do I think that pregnancy controls a woman's destiny? Does it have to?
- Do I believe that my freedom rests in controlling my childbearing? What does "control" mean?
- Do I think that going through one pregnancy will mean that I will go through many more?
- Do I believe that society wants to keep women "poor, barefoot, and pregnant"? Is it possible to be pregnant while rejecting the second-class role of women?
- Am I a feminist? How do I define feminism?
- Does a feminist bow to society's pressure or strive to change society?
- Can a true feminist give birth to her baby while working to make her own future into what she wants it to be? Will such a woman's actions pave the way for other women to have their babies without ruining their futures?
- How liberated or equal am I if I can have a good future only by denying my pregnancy? Is this liberation? Or am I still enslaved to the double standard that says a man can sow his wild oats but a woman better not get caught?
- Will I, by having my baby and refusing to compromise my future, help end the double standard?

CHANGES

- What do I think of changes? Do I hate or fear change? Do I like the excitement of change?

- What would be my reaction if I were fired from my job? Suppose I were evicted from my home? How would I feel if a ten-ton truck ran over my car while I was shopping? What do my answers tell me about my attitude toward change?

Fears for Yourself

- What changes are bothering me, in addition to those discussed earlier?
- Am I afraid of nausea, exhaustion, or other pregnancy discomforts? Do I know that a doctor can help alleviate these common problems?
- Am I afraid that pregnancy will change my lifestyle? Do I know that pregnancy need not stop me from doing just about anything that I am doing now?
- Do I think that pregnancy will make me ugly, sluggish, or dull? Can I break my stereotype of the pregnant, dowdy woman sitting around doing nothing, waiting for her baby to be born?
- Have I ever seen a vibrant, energetic, beautiful pregnant woman? Do I think that such a woman could exist? How can I be one?
- Do I think that giving birth requires a long recuperation? Do I know that most women need only a few weeks at most to recover from giving birth?
- What is my company's maternity leave?
- Am I afraid of giving birth? Why? Did I hear or read horror stories about childbirth? Did I hear stories about what my parents "went through" to have me?
- Can I read some books or take a hospital course and confront my fears?

NEGATIVE THOUGHTS ABOUT YOUR BABY

- Am I repulsed by the thought of a baby growing in my body? Do I feel like a host to a parasite? Why do I have this repulsion? Would a counselor or psychologist help me uncover the basis of my disgust?
- Did my mother (or someone else) tell me that I was a "mistake" or the result of failed birth control? Have her words influenced me against this baby I didn't plan?
- Do I see the world as spinning toward destruction?
- Do I think I am foolish for having a child now?
- What good things am I missing in the world?
- Do I think my child might help improve the world?
- Would I want my child to experience no change, no suffering in life? Since I know that every life experiences both, have I decided not to have a child to spare that child pain?
- Have I felt that the pain in my own life far overshadowed the joy?
- How can I change my own future into something brighter than the past? Can I do the same for my baby?

UNEASE ABOUT OTHERS

- Do I know the phone number and address of my local PREGNANCY AIDgency?
- Am I afraid a volunteer will persuade me to do something I don't want to do?
- Am I embarrassed to seek help?
- Do I hate revealing my intimate thoughts and concerns? Do I fear being hurt should I do so?
- Why do I think a PREGNANCY AIDgency would misunderstand me when its primary work is with women in pregnancy crisis?
- Am I too proud to admit that someone else may offer new insights into my problems?
- Do I have any prejudices against PREGNANCY AIDgencies? Against other counselors? What are these prejudices? Are they valid?

- What is keeping me from having my baby?
- Am I experiencing any crisis other than the pregnancy?
- Is some person or some ideal pressuring me to abort?
- Do I think that my lifestyle is in jeopardy if I continue my pregnancy?
- If I think that my pregnancy will destroy my future, what does that tell me about the control I have over my life?
- How will this pregnancy redirect my life? What barriers do I see? Are these barriers mainly in my mind? Can they be overcome? Am I a strong enough person to overcome them?

EVALUATING YOUR ANSWERS

- Perhaps you learned something by answering these questions. How do you feel about yourself now? About your answers?
- Have you surprised yourself, uncovered hidden motives, relived painful memories?
- How can what you have learned help you to have your baby? To plan for your own future? For your baby's future?

Appendix E

CHOOSING PROFESSIONAL CARE

Many women simply call a physician or other professional and use that person throughout their pregnancy. If you want a choice in the type of person who treats you, and in the type of care and birth experience you'll have, use the questions in this Appendix. Some questions are for you to answer after you meet with a professional. These questions will help you understand what qualities you are looking for in a professional and what type of treatment you desire. Other questions are for the professional to answer in your presence, so that you will know exactly what options you're being offered.

Discuss your choice of professionals and your treatment options with a counselor or confidant before making a decision. You have a right to understand your treatment and to make choices for yourself and your baby. Utilize that right.

CHOOSING PROFESSIONALS

Choose professionals who will support your decision to give birth. After speaking to professionals, analyze what you've heard. Here are some questions to consider.

Professional's Views on Abortion

- Does this person know that abortion is hardly ever medically necessary?
- Do you sense respect for your decision to give birth?
- Does the person have a casual attitude toward abortion? Or does the individual recognize that abortion deeply affects many women?

Professional's Views on Your Right to Seek and Understand Treatment

- What is the person's reaction if you say that you might seek a second opinion?
- Is the professional willing to explain side effects and complications of and reasons for procedures, drugs, and tests? How about explaining unfamiliar terms? Or do you hear that you wouldn't understand or don't need to know? Do you feel "talked down to"?
- Does this person speak slowly? Clearly? Intelligently? Truthfully? Do you think some information is being withheld or misstated?
- If you or your child is facing a medical difficulty, does your doctor schedule tests to evaluate the problem, or does the doctor make diagnoses and sweeping statements without testing?
- Does your doctor know about recent advances in medical technology? Is your doctor willing to find out?
- Will this doctor refer you to another doctor or to another hospital if necessary?
- If you ask questions, express preferences, or show feelings, does this person treat you like an intelligent human being?
- Do you feel comfortable with this person? Or would you rather switch?

Other Considerations

- How does the professional react when discussing payment?
- Will insurance pay for your medical expenses?
- Will the office file any necessary forms for payment or will you have to do it? Will you have to pay first and file forms later to be reimbursed?
- Will a lawyer discuss and evaluate every option?
- Does a lawyer suggest manipulating the truth in court? Where might this lead?
- Is a psychologist patient and compassionate, willing to let you "talk it out," or do you feel hurried, pressured, or misunderstood?
- Does a psychologist seem too quick to prescribe drugs?
- Is a psychologist or assistant available to talk in emergencies?

MAKING A CHOICE

Review your answers to the above questions. Choose a professional who explains procedures, gives you options and statistics, and respects your right to give birth. Find one who seems knowledgeable, flexible, and straightforward. You need to be able to talk to and trust professionals so that you will have a good pregnancy and birth experience.

PLANNING YOUR LABOR AND DELIVERY

You have many choices for labor and delivery. Today you can have a totally medicated birth during which you know nothing until you recover from general anesthesia, or you can have a totally natural birth in which you give birth squatting or in water and never have an episiotomy, enema, or medication. Or you can have anything in between. It's important to know that, today, you can choose the birth experience that's best for you.

Speak to other mothers who have recently given birth. Ask your hospital what birth options it offers. Read books on childbirth options. Attend childbirth classes. Get an idea of the type of birth experience you'd like and write it down. Then discuss your plan and the following questions with your doctor or midwife. Also discuss the recommendations in the "Pregnant Patient's Bill of Rights" and the "Pregnant Patient's Responsibilities," as referred to in Chapter Three. Choose a doctor or midwife who will give you the plan you want while also keeping in mind what is safest and most comfortable for you and your baby.

Questions About Choosing a Birth Experience

- What types of childbirth options do you offer?
- What is your opinion of my childbirth plan?
- Can you refer me to other women who have had a birth experience similar to the one I'd like?
- Where can I learn about natural childbirth? Can you refer me to natural childbirth classes? What books on natural childbirth do you recommend?
- Where can I learn about home birth? What are the advantages and disadvantages of home birth? What is your experience with home birth? Considering my proximity to a hospital in case of an emergency, would you consider home birth a good option for me?
- What can you tell me about a medicated birth? What medications are used? Why? Which can I request? If I want to refuse medications, can I do so?
- Do you anticipate a Cesarean section for me? Do you recommend a local or general anesthetic? Why?
- Will a partner, relative, or friend be with me in labor and delivery?

Questions About Labor and Delivery

- How long can I safely stay at home during early labor? When should I go to the hospital? How frequent and how long should my contractions be before I call you? What other signs of labor should I look for?
- What can I bring to the hospital to occupy my mind during early labor? How about card games, books, knitting, or mending? Can I watch television? Is one available?
- What can I eat or drink during labor? Can I suck on fruit juice ice cubes or lick lollipops to give me both liquid and energy? Do I have to bring these from home? Will the hospital supply them?
- How much monitoring during labor can I expect? What examinations will I receive? What devices will be used? Can I refuse these? What if I do?
- Must I spend my entire labor lying on a delivery table, strapped to monitors? What if I refuse to do this? Can I walk during labor or do whatever else seems more comfortable?
- Will you, as doctor or midwife, induce labor? Why? What tests will you do to make sure that induction is medically necessary? Can I refuse induction? What might happen if I do? Is induced labor more difficult for me to manage, more painful? Might it be ineffective and result in a Cesarean section? Can I safely wait for labor to begin or progress naturally?
- Can I try a specific birth technique or position? How about giving birth while in a squatting position? Sitting in a birthing chair? Lying in a delivery room? Resting in a birthing room? Supported in a water bath? Do I have to have an episiotomy? A pubic shave? An enema?

Questions About Procedures After Your Baby Is Born

- What will happen to my baby upon birth?
- Which of these can I request or refuse for my baby? A dim, quiet birthing room? A warm bath after birth? Breastfeeding immediately after birth? Rooming-in totally from birth on? Circumcision? Bottle-feeding? Breastfeeding? What are the advantages and disadvantages of each choice?
- Who can visit me in the hospital? My spouse? Children? Relatives? Can they see the baby?
- When can I go home from the hospital? Hours after birth? A day later? In a few days?
- Will insurance pay for a person to help me in my home for a few days after I give birth?

A Good Plan

Together with your doctor or midwife, confirm your plan for labor and delivery. Then write it down. A few weeks before your due date, give a copy of your plan to your doctor or midwife and to the hospital, if you will be giving birth there. Doing so will increase your chances of having the birth experience you prefer.

Have copies of the plan with you when you actually go into labor. Hand the copies out again to your caregivers and hospital. This will remind everyone of what you've already planned, and your caregivers will more likely respect your choices when you are actually giving birth.

MEDICAL DIFFICULTIES

When you or your baby faces medical difficulties, you have a right to complete information. Take this book along with you when you visit your doctor. Discuss with your physician the "Pregnant Patient's Bill of Rights" and the "Pregnant Patient's Responsibilities," referred to in Chapter Three. Does your physician agree with these documents?

Also ask your doctor any of the following questions that fit your circumstances. You may adapt some questions or think of others. Jot these down and ask. Write down the answers to these questions as you discuss them with your doctor, or tape-record the conversation so that you have an accurate account.

General Questions to Ask About Medical Difficulties

- Exactly how is this pregnancy going to affect me or my baby? What specific problems do you foresee?
- What is the probability, in percentages, of one of us developing one of these problems? May I see the source of your information?
- What tests can determine if these problems are actually present? Do you recommend these tests?
- How much do these tests cost? Will my insurance pay for them?
- If I have these tests, what is the margin of safety, given in percentages, for me and my baby? What risks, if any, do my baby and I face from these tests? What is the percentage of risk? The severity of risk?
- How accurate are these tests, in percentages? What is the possibility of error?
- Can these tests be done in this area? If not, where?
- May I see your medical literature on this type of testing?
- Would you recommend this testing if I plan to continue my pregnancy, no matter what the test reveals?
- What causes these problems? Did my partner or I do anything to cause these problems? Can we do anything to keep them from getting worse or from happening again?
- Is there any treatment for these problems? What? How costly is it? Will insurance cover it?
- How is treatment done? When must treatment begin? Is there any reason why treatment must be done at the time you suggest? Is it possible to wait? How long?
- What is the probability of success in treating these problems, given in percentages? Are there alternate treatments? What are their success rates?
- May I see your literature on the treatment of this problem?
- Can you refer me to other women who have faced these problems? Are there any local or national support groups for women facing these problems? How can I contact these groups?

Questions to Ask if You Face Your Own Possible Death

- Are you saying that I will definitely die if I have this baby? If so, why? If not, then what medical problems do you think I will have?
- Are you saying that you expect definite, life-threatening medical problems with this pregnancy or are you saying that there *might* be medical problems?
- What is your estimate of risk?
- What percentage of women with my condition have experienced these problems?
- What is the range of severity of these problems?
- Can I deliver my baby early, then receive more aggressive treatment?
- Are you concerned that I will be unable to properly care for my baby because of my condition? Is this why you are suggesting abortion?
- May I see literature on pregnancy among women with my condition?

Questions to Ask if You Have a Baby With Special Needs or Health Problems

- If prenatal tests indicate that my unborn child has special needs or health problems, can you tell how severe these problems will be? Could you refer me to a parent or institution that cares for children with these needs? Could I visit these children?

- Does my child need surgery or medication? What type? How much? What does this cost? Will insurance pay for the treatments?
- Do you know of anyone who has made an adoption plan for a child such as mine?
- If you cannot refer me to anyone, can you suggest someone I can call for a referral?
- If my child experiences a medical crisis either before or after birth, will you aggressively treat the problem?
- Will you deny treatment to my child that other children would receive? Why or why not?
- Can you give me specific examples of how you have treated children with this problem either before or after birth?
- If both my baby and I have medical difficulties, will you treat my unborn child the same way you would have if I were healthy?
- Will you fully discuss with me all treatment or nontreatment options for my child?
- If my child has a fatal abnormality or a terminal illness, will you respect my wishes to give my child the best possible chance of living? Will you allow death to occur naturally when medical science can do no more to help my baby?

Questions to Ask if Your Baby Dies

- What makes you certain that my baby has died?
- What prenatal tests can I have to confirm that my baby has died?
- Should I have a pregnancy test that measures the level of pregnancy hormones? Is my hormonal level at or far below normal limits? What does this mean?
- What could have caused my baby to die? A genetic condition? Environmental hazard? Something I did or did not do? Is there any way to prevent this from happening in another pregnancy?
- Is this cramping normal?
- How long will the bleeding last? Why is the blood so bright? Should these blood clots concern me?
- Why do I still have a positive pregnancy test if I have all this bleeding?
- Should I rest?
- Will I hemorrhage?
- Can I get an infection?
- What should I do with the pregnancy tissue?
- Do I need any surgical procedures? Why? Please describe these procedures in detail. Do you suggest that I be awake or asleep for these? What are the advantages and disadvantages of either option?
- Would you suggest an autopsy for my baby? How might I arrange for one?
- May I have my baby's body for burial?
- When can I resume sexual relations?
- When can I get pregnant again?
- Will this pregnancy loss happen again? What can I do to avoid another pregnancy loss?

Evaluating What You Hear

Review your doctor's answers before making any decisions. Also consult literature on the topic and strongly consider obtaining a second and third opinion before choosing treatment. With a confidant or counselor, separate feelings from facts before deciding what to do.

Appendix F

EVALUATING LIFESTYLE OPTIONS

You are facing many decisions and you want to decide well. In making any decision, first you must get all the facts. Then you must compare the choices by considering the facts. Finally, you must decide and then take the responsibility for your choice.

Obviously, you can make only one choice of the several you have. For example, if you choose to parent your baby, you are not choosing adoption (although you can change your mind later and then choose it). If you don't choose well initially, you can always choose again, but you may have experienced much stress and pain by making a wrong choice and then correcting it. This Appendix should help you choose wisely the first time.

First decide which decisions you must make. Not every section of this Appendix will apply to your own situation, but some sections will. Discuss your answers to the questions in those sections with a counselor or your confidant. Based on your answers, what is the best choice for you and your baby?

If you don't have a clear-cut choice, try writing down the good and bad aspects of each choice you have. Which choice will result in the most good? Perhaps that is the choice you should make.

DECIDING WHETHER TO CONTINUE YOUR EDUCATION OR CAREER

You may have difficulty choosing between your education or career and motherhood, or you may want to have both simultaneously. Depending upon your age and situation, discuss the following questions with a vocational counselor or your confidant, partner, or parents or guardians.

Career? Education? Motherhood?

- How do I feel about continuing my education or career and about motherhood? Would I want to have both? Would I want to choose one and not the other? Why do I feel this way?
- What is my attitude toward career mothers or student mothers?
- Can I financially afford to parent a child? Why or why not? How can I better manage my finances to make room for a baby? Would a financial consultant help?
- Can I afford the time to parent a baby now? Do I have take-home assignments regularly? Can I do these if I am parenting? Who can watch my baby while I do this take-home work?
- How do I feel about day care? About a baby sitter in my home? Where do my feelings originate? How would I find day care or a sitter whom I could really trust? Through newspaper ads? Through a friend? Through a religious institution? Through my family?
- If I want to keep my baby with me while working, can I hire a baby sitter to come to work with me?

- Does my company, place of work, or educational institution have a child care center? Should I suggest beginning one? How would my company or educational institution react?
- If I want to be a full-time mom, how will I feel about giving up my career or education for a few years? Am I afraid that I would be bored, unfulfilled, or stifled?
- If I am thinking about dropping out of high school or college to parent my baby, am I making a good choice? What would be the consequences of my not having a diploma? Would I ever go back to school to finish my education? Why or why not? Does my education matter? Why?
- Do I feel ignorant of child care? Do I think I would do a bad job? How can I learn the art of mothering? Through books? Parenting courses? Advice of friends?
- How would my husband or boyfriend feel about my combining a career or education with motherhood? How would he feel if I gave up one for the other? Do I care how he feels?
- If I am thinking of giving up my job to parent my child, where will I get the money I need? Can I use government assistance? Can my partner support the two of us and the baby on one salary? Will we have to adjust our lifestyle? How? How will both of us feel about that?
- How can I parent my baby and maintain my career or continue my education? Is adoption better? How do I feel about each option?

Making A Wise Choice

Choose the option that will give you the most satisfaction and the least stress in the long run. You may have to make some trade-offs for a while in order to achieve your desired long-term goals.

CHOOSING WHETHER OR NOT TO MARRY

If you're deciding whether or not to marry either your baby's father or another man, consider these questions. Marriage is a big commitment. Think carefully before choosing it.

Your Reasons for Considering Marriage

Why am I considering marriage?

- Because I'm pregnant?
- To give my baby a name?
- Because I think it's the proper thing to do?
- Because someone else wants me to?
- So that other people won't talk about me?
- Because I want to feel needed and worthwhile?
- For companionship?
- Are any of these good enough reasons for marriage?
- Would I be considering marriage if I were not pregnant?
- Why should someone be getting married?
- Do I love this man enough to want to spend my whole life with him?

"Costs" of Marriage

- Am I willing to give up my freedom to be married now?
- Will marriage to this man cause me to abandon my educational or career goals? Why? How does this make me feel?
- Am I willing to adjust my lifestyle to accommodate this man and marriage?

- Am I ready to take on the responsibility of caring for myself, my baby, and this man as well?
- Is this man ready to give himself totally to the care of his child and to me as his wife? Will he do this forever or will he lose interest? Will I lose interest in him?
- Do I think this marriage will last? Will we work to make it last?

Understanding the Man You Are Considering Marrying

- Is this man willing to let me be my own person or does he want to control me?
- Does he want me to baby him or to wait on him?
- Who does this man view as the authority in the family?
- What kind of a man is he? Is he someone I can love, trust, and admire?
- Can I confide in him?
- Is he mature enough to be a husband and a dad? Will he change in the future?
- Does he still have a lot of growing up to do?
- Do I think I can change this man after marriage? What if I can't? Can I accept him then?
- What faults does this man have? Can I accept and live with them?
- Does this man treat me the same when we are alone as when we are with his friends and family?
- Can I get along with this man's friends and family? Can he get along with mine?
- How well do we communicate? Can we share feelings?
- How much do we argue? Does one person always give in to the other?
- Has this man ever physically or emotionally abused me?
- Does he have a jealous nature?
- Does he have a drug or alcohol problem?
- Does he cheat on me?
- What kind of family background does he have? How much will it influence the type of husband and father he will be?

Practical Considerations

- If I marry this man, will we have the finances and the maturity to make this marriage work?
- Who is going to get a job? One or both of us?
- What happens after the baby comes? Will I keep my job or stay home? How will that work out? Do I like this arrangement?
- Will we share finances? Can we budget?
- Will we share household tasks?
- How will we delegate job responsibilities in the home?
- Can we enjoy recreation, hobbies, and vacations together? Are our interests radically different?
- Is religion important to one or both of us? Do we have similar beliefs?
- If we have different religious beliefs, will one of us try to "convert" the other?
- How will we handle religion with our children?
- Do we agree on the number of children we want to have?
- Will we share parenting responsibilities?
- What is our philosophy of child rearing? Of motherhood? Fatherhood?
- Is sex the most important aspect of our relationship? Should it be?
- What is this man's view of sexual intimacy?
- How often will he want to have intercourse? Am I comfortable with this?
- What future goals does this man have? How does he want to meet them? Do I agree?

To Marry or Not?

Think carefully about how you answered these questions. Ask someone who knows this man well to answer the questions also. Do your answers match the other person's? What have you learned about the man you are considering for a husband? Is he good husband and parent material? Do you both have similar views? Do you have solid reasons for wanting to marry now?

If you are not sure whether you should marry, wait. Your hesitation is an indication that you have doubts. Rethink your decision and marry only when you're sure. Otherwise, you may be headed for failure. As someone commented, "It's better to be single than to be married to the wrong person."

EVALUATING AN AFFAIR

If you are involved in an affair, it means that either you or your lover is committed to someone else. One, or both of you have two or more intimate relationships at the same time. For example, you or your lover may be married to, engaged to, or living with someone else. No matter which of you has committed yourself to another relationship, you are both involved in an affair.

The questions in this section will help you understand why you are involved in an affair and the consequences of continuing. They will also help you decide if you wish to remain with either of your lovers. Often people who know you or your lover, or both of you, can help you logically evaluate an affair. Discuss the questions in this section with a few of these people. Use your head as well as your heart in making a decision. You may be madly in love with a certain man, but you should ask yourself whether it is wise to continue the relationship.

Why?

- Why did you begin an affair? Were you bored? Abused? Disgusted? Alone? Was your sex life unfulfilling? Did you want excitement? Did you need financial support?
- Did you fall in love unintentionally?
- What does your lover supply that no one else does?
- What is especially attractive about your lover?

If He Is Married

- Are you comfortable with never being seen with this married man in public, never calling him at home, having to be available to him whenever he wants?
- Why did he tell you he loves you?
- What has he told you about his wife? Do you believe him? Should you?
- If you are single, have you taken yourself out of circulation to be involved with a married man? Who might you be missing?
- Do you really believe this man will someday marry you?
- Have you ever thought that a man who cheats on his wife will probably someday cheat on you? How do you feel about that?

If You Are in an Uncommitted Relationship

- Have either you or your lover made no commitments to each other? Are you comfortable with this?
- Is your lover involved with other women? Do you know for sure?
- Can you accept your lover's probable sexual involvement with others?
- Can you handle the probable end of your relationship(s) at some future time?

- Should you end your relationship(s) now? Keep one or both?
- Do you want to parent your baby in this uncommitted situation?
- Do you want to risk disease from a man who may be bed hopping? How can you protect your health if you continue sexual activity with this lover?
- Is your baby's father going to marry you or make a commitment to you? When?
- If he is married or committed to someone else, is he going to divorce his wife or sever his other relationship? When? Will he set a date and keep it?
- Do you want to continue your relationship with this man, with you always being the other woman?

If You Have Two Lovers

- Which man, of your two lovers, do you really "love"? Which one loves you? How can you tell?
- Which man is legally, emotionally, and financially ready to support you? To support your plans for your baby? Will one or both men pressure you to abort?
- Should you end one relationship and maintain the other? Should you end both relationships?
- What are the advantages of each decision? The disadvantages?
- How will both lovers react to you and to your baby?
- If you end a relationship, could a lover endanger you?
- Do you *have* to maintain a certain relationship? Why? If you wish to break free of this relationship, what help do you need?
- Do you need legal counsel? Police protection? A restraining order against one lover so that he faces arrest if he harasses or threatens to harm you?

Complications

- What complications of your affair, besides pregnancy, are you facing? Guilt? Deception? Fear of discovery? Organizational difficulties in maintaining two relationships? Mistrust? Other unpleasant consequences?
- Do you want to preserve two relationships? Should you?
- Must you keep each man ignorant of the other? Of the pregnancy? How can you do this and still give birth?
- Will information in Chapter Two, on keeping your pregnancy a secret, help you?
- Is there any way one man will know *for certain* that your baby could *never* be his? Do you want to continue your relationship with this man?
- Can you anticipate this man's reaction to your affair? To your pregnancy? To you? To your baby?
- Will family counseling help you both?
- Do you need to keep this pregnancy hidden?
- Will you need to live elsewhere for a while?
- Do you want to parent this child?
- Must you make an adoption plan?
- What other arrangements can you make?

Revealing Your Affair

- Is your affair over, really over?
- Does anyone know about your affair? Suspect it? Who? Will they tell? Can they *prove* you've had an affair? Would it be your word against theirs? Who would people believe?
- Can you counteract gossip? Will gossip force you to admit your affair?
- Does your original lover suspect your affair? Will he, ever?

- Is there a possibility, even a small one, that the baby could be his? If so, should you reveal your affair?
- What good will come to you if you admit that you've had an affair? Will you release fear or guilt? What good will your admission do for your lover?
- Will admitting your affair strengthen your relationship? How?
- If a man suspects the child is not his, how will he feel toward the child? Toward you? Himself? Your relationship?
- What good will come to your family if you tell of your affair?
- Are you afraid to reveal your affair? What reaction can you expect if you do?
- Can you regain your lover's trust if you admit to having an affair?
- Is it better to confide in a member of the clergy or counselor and not to your lover?
- Do you want to continue your relationship with your baby's father? Does he know about your original lover? Should you tell him if he doesn't know?

Deciding What to Do About an Affair

Decide what to do about an affair before making any plans for your baby. Your plans for the baby might change if your relationships change. So work on the relationships first.

Discussing your answers to these questions with someone else may help you see your affair in a clearer light. Perhaps you will decide to end one relationship or both. Do what will bring the best results in the long run, even though it may cause some temporary pain.

EVALUATING INDIVIDUAL OR GROUP PRESSURE

An individual or group may exercise control over your decisions and behaviors. You may never have thought of evaluating the influence others have on you. Now you may be told what to do about your pregnancy or your baby. Before blindly following the advice of others, evaluate your situation.

Choose the section or sections below that apply to your situation. Discuss your answers to these questions with someone who is not also influenced by the group or individual. This person might be a counselor, confidant, or member of the clergy. Your answers to these questions may help you determine the degree of pressure a person or group is exerting on you and what you should do about it.

Questions to Ask if Someone Is Predicting Your Future

- Is this person giving me concrete, specific advice or general information?
- How many of the "predictions" are based on information I have already revealed?
- Is this person well versed in human behavior?
- Can this person predict what I will probably think and do by carefully observing me and by asking leading questions? Is this really foreseeing the future or is it predicting how I would probably act? Is it predicting the types of situations that someone like me is likely to encounter?
- Has this person always been accurate in directing me? Has some advice gone wrong?
- If something has not turned out as predicted, did this individual have a "reason" for what happened? Could this reason have been made up after the prediction failed?
- Is the future, as told to me, so vague or given in such symbolic terms that almost anything that happens can be said to have happened as was predicted?
- Does this person hold a position of decision making in the community, such as a council member, judge, or board member, in which power to foresee the future would be invaluable? If not, why not?

Questions to Ask if You Feel "Bound" to an Individual

- Do I owe this person money? How much? Have I paid this person in the past? How much? What services am I paying for?
- Am I in "financial bondage" to this person?
- Do I need this person to supply me with the lifestyle I am used to having?
- What was my life like before I met this person?
- Has this person helped me to become more independent? How?
- Have I leaned on this person as an emotional crutch for decision making?
- Do I feel in control or do I feel controlled?
- Do I need confidence in making my own decisions? Is this person inspiring such confidence or not?
- Is it time to break away from this person?

Questions to Ask if You Feel "Bound" to a Group

- What do I like about this group? Why am I a part of this group? What's in it for me?
- Do I have any addictions that the group fosters? Do I want to give them up? Why or why not?
- Does this group manipulate, humiliate, or degrade me? How do I feel about this? How do I feel about myself? Why?
- What pressures does this group put on me?
- Does the group control its members? How?
- Do group members have to conform?
- Am I afraid of this group?
- Have I seen this group harm others?
- Does this group discourage professional medical care? Why? Is this safe for me? For my baby?
- Does this group encourage abortion, child abuse, or severe discipline of children?
- Am I in emotional, financial, or physical bondage to this group?
- Have I been brainwashed?
- Do I have the freedom to leave the group or is someone always with me?
- How does this group treat children born to group members?
- Does someone have plans for my child? What are they? Do I believe that they will carry these out?
- Do I know my child's father? Am I afraid of him? Is he a group member? How does this affect me?
- Am I pregnant willingly or have I been raped?
- Am I comfortable with everything that goes on in this group? What bothers me?
- Would this group accept my pregnancy? My child? Why or why not?
- Can I leave this group freely? What will happen if I try to go?

Taking Control Yourself

If your answers to these questions alarm you, you may consider leaving the controlling group or individual. Remember, no one person or group should control your life or your baby's. You have free will. You can make choices and so can your baby, in time. Call the police, a women's resource center, counseling centers, a member of the clergy, or PREGNANCY AIDgencies if you need help. Appendix H lists additional agencies to consult.

Appendix G

PARENTING CHOICES

In making decisions about parenting your baby, it's best to talk to people who are in situations similar to yours but who have made different choices. Speak to birth parents—those who are parenting their children and those who have made an adoption plan. Talk to an adoption consultant and to an instructor of parenting classes. If your child has special needs or a terminal illness, also speak to people in charge of adoptive, group, or institutional homes for such children.

Discuss with these people the questions in this Appendix. How would they answer? Use their guidance and your own answers to these questions to make the parenting choice that's right for you.

CHOOSING BETWEEN PARENTING, ADOPTION, OR ANOTHER PARENTING PLAN

You can choose whether to parent your baby. Here are several questions to consider. List the good and bad points about adoption and parenting. Discuss your answers with an adoption consultant and confidant. Which list is longer? Which option is wisest for you?

Ulterior Motives

- Am I keeping this baby so that I can move out on my own? Am I ready to live on my own with my baby?
- How easy will it be to manage a home and a baby myself? Can I get someone to help me?
- Am I keeping this baby to take away my loneliness? Will the baby really make me feel less lonely?
- Do I know what it is like to live with a baby full-time, communicating on a baby's level? Will this childish exchange really take away my loneliness?
- Am I keeping this baby so that people will think I'm mature? Am I really mature?
- Will I actually be any more grown up when the baby is born than I am now?
- Am I keeping this baby so that the baby's father will love me more or marry me?
- Do I think the baby's father will come around to see the baby?
- Will I still want my baby if the baby's father deserts me?
- Am I keeping this baby because others think I should? What do I think?
- Do I feel unloved?
- Do I love myself?
- Am I keeping this baby so that my baby will love me?
- Do I think that a baby will make me feel important?

Misunderstandings About Adoption

- Do I think that a child belongs with his birth mother?
- Do I have negative thoughts about women who make adoption plans for their children?
- Do I have negative ideas about adopted children?
- Am I keeping my baby because I do not understand adoption or because, emotionally, I don't like the idea? Are my emotions based on fact?
- Where can I obtain information about modern adoption?
- Am I keeping this baby because I have fears about adoptive families? What causes these fears?
- Do I fear that an adoptive family will abuse my child? Can someone relieve these fears?
- Do I know how carefully an adoption agency chooses adoptive families?
- Am I afraid to choose adoption because I can't imagine "giving up" my child?
- Would I always wonder how my child was doing?
- Do I know that I can learn how my adopted child is doing?
- Do I know that I might be able to correspond with the adoptive family and even visit my child?
- How can I find out what information I can have about my growing child?
- Am I keeping my child because I am married and because I never heard of a married woman making an adoption plan?
- Where can I learn about adoption for children of married women?
- If I choose adoption, would I feel like a failure as a wife or mother? Why would I feel this way? Should I feel this way?
- Do I know a family that might adopt my child? Could I find one by asking family or friends?

Understanding Other Parenting Options

- Have I considered other parenting options?
- What do I think of temporary foster care (no more than a year at most)? Would this help me? How?
- Would parenting by a relative work? Would I want to make this person my child's legal guardian?
- Is a group home or institution a good choice for my child? Why? Where can I locate a good home?

Parenting Responsibilities

- Even though I like children, am I ready to have one full-time at this time of my life? Why or why not?
- What freedom do I have now? Am I ready to give up this freedom?
- When my friends go out, will I want to stay home with my child?
- Will I resent the amount of time the baby requires and the demands that this baby will make on me?
- Am I a patient person?
- Do I live in a calm, secure household?
- Would my child be in danger of abuse?
- How will I react when my child gets sick? What if the sickness lasts a long time?
- How will I handle a difficult-to-raise or strong-willed child?
- Is my partner patient? Will he be a good, loving dad?
- If my partner and I are not married, are we planning marriage? When? Do I want to raise my child with a man to whom I'm not married?
- How much do I love my baby?

- Am I willing to put my child's interests and needs before my own?
- Can I adjust emotionally to the time, sacrifice, and interrupted lifestyle that accompany raising a baby?
- Do I know how to raise a baby? Do I want to learn? Where can I learn?
- Can I handle my child as a toddler, young child, adolescent, teen?
- Do I understand that I will actively parent for eighteen years at least and then still be parenting for a lifetime?
- Am I ready, willing, and able to devote my life to this baby?

Parenting Philosophy

- How do I think a parent should raise a child?
- What values, morals, and character traits do I hope to instill in my child? Can I discuss child rearing with someone or read some books on parenting?
- What mistakes did my parents make in raising me? How can I avoid making these mistakes?
- Can I lovingly discipline my baby? How?
- How will I handle my child when I lose my temper?

Facing Changes

- What are my plans for the future? Will raising my baby change those plans? How? How do I feel about that?
- Will having to change my plans eventually hurt both me and my baby? Will I resent my child for having caused me to change my plans?
- Can I raise my baby and still follow my plans for the future? How? Who will help me?
- How do I feel about having a larger family than I planned?
- How do I feel about returning to the ''baby routine''?
- Can I think of creative ways to bring my baby into a family of older children?

Emotional Adjustments

- If I am pregnant due to an affair or to rape, am I comfortable raising a baby who is not my lover's?
- Will I eventually look forward to having and raising a baby even though I hadn't planned on parenting now?
- Do I have a good sense of humor?
- If I'm expecting another child and already have one or more small children, will a ''light heart and merry spirit'' help me raise several small children all at the same time?
- Will my determination help me raise a child even though my mental or physical health may not be good?
- Will I love a child of either sex equally?
- Can I lovingly raise my divorced husband's baby?
- Can I parent my deceased husband's baby?
- Can I love a child of a man I dislike?

Dealing With Others

- Are others pressuring me to make a certain parenting decision? Who? Why are they pressuring me? What can I say or do to deal with this pressure?
- How can I tactfully deal with comments that imply that I am ''overpopulating'' by having too many children?
- How will I handle the advice, support, or meddling of family and friends?
- What will be my reaction if someone tells me that parenting my baby or choosing adoption is going to be the biggest mistake of my life?

- If I am a single mother, what will I say if people ask about my baby's father? Will I resent their questions?
- Can I handle prying questions tactfully while maintaining privacy?
- What will I tell my child about the birth father?
- Do I think that parenting my baby may make it more difficult for me to get married later?
- What will I tell future boyfriends about my child?
- Can I confide in someone when I have problems?
- Who will help me when I need a break from child rearing? Is anyone available to babysit? Will I have to pay this person? How much?
- What type of relationship will I have with my parents or other relatives if I parent my baby? Will they support my decision? Will they help me?

Practical Considerations

- Am I living in an "adults only" housing complex? If I parent my child, how difficult will it be to find other housing? Will I resent moving? Can I afford other housing?
- Do I qualify for housing assistance?
- Do I need extra room for the baby?
- How do I feel about moving to a larger home or apartment or adding on to my current home?
- How will I rework a job schedule or a family routine?
- Will I need to adjust career or educational goals? How will parenting my baby affect my career or education?
- What adjustments must I make after the baby is born? Will these involve day care arrangements? Sitters? A nanny? Am I emotionally prepared to make these adjustments? If not, can I change my attitude?
- What expenses will I have if I parent my child? Will I have enough money? Can I adjust my finances? If not, how can I manage?
- Can I apply for government aid?
- Can I get an additional job?
- Will someone help me financially? Who?
- Will I have to do without some things to buy what my baby needs?
- Can a financial planner help me? Where can I find a financial planner?
- What baby furniture, baby clothing, and other items will I need? How will I get them? Can I get some from a PREGNANCY AIDgency, from family or friends, or inexpensively at garage sales or thrift shops? What government agency can I contact to be sure that secondhand items meet current safety standards?
- Do I plan to bottle-feed or breastfeed my baby? How will I be able to do this?
- If I plan to breastfeed, is there a breastfeeding support group nearby for advice and support?
- How will my feeding plans affect other areas of my life such as job, education, and recreation?

Choosing a Parenting Plan

Your choice of a parenting plan will affect you, your baby, and many others. Others affected might include your husband, children, parents, neighbors, and friends or the adoptive family and its extended family and social circle. Think through your plan frequently. Brainstorm some alternate plans, even if you don't think you'd ever follow them, just to see how you feel about them. Sometimes what we once felt we'd never consider seems more reasonable with time.

Use your confidant to help you formulate a plan that will work. The plan will be tailor-made for you. If one plan does not obviously seem to be the best, review your options again with a counselor or confidant. If you still cannot make a choice, placing your baby in foster care can give you a few months more to decide. Choose a plan that will help both you and your baby to become all you were both meant to be.

PARENTING THE CHILD WITH SPECIAL NEEDS OR A TERMINAL ILLNESS

If you are considering parenting a child with special needs or a terminal illness, use the previous questions as well as these to make a choice. Answering the previous questions can help you discover why you are considering a certain parenting option. The questions in this section will help you uncover the facts about parenting your child.

Answer the questions here in consultation with a teacher, doctor, or caseworker who has experience with children similar to your own child. Write down the answers to the questions and discuss them with your partner or confidant. Speak to parents of other children whose problems are similar to those of your child, and see how they handled the difficulties that arose. Use their input as well as your own answers to make some informed choices.

Practical Considerations

- What needs does my child have?
- What is the medical prognosis?
- What treatments or special equipment does my child need?
- What experimental treatments or equipment might I try?
- Does my child require hospitalization or surgery? Might surgery improve my child's physical appearance?
- What other medical services does my child need? Are these available in my area? If not, where?
- Can someone design a piece of equipment to help my child? Who?
- Can I obtain, fit into my home, and learn to use my child's equipment?
- Is my house suitable in design and layout for a child with a physical or motor problem?

Financial Considerations

- What will my child's care and equipment cost? Can I afford it?
- Will insurance pay some expenses? Which ones?
- Will either my partner or I have to get a second job to pay for these expenses?
- Can anyone raise funds, donate money, or write a loan to help? Who?

Emotional Considerations

- What might my life with this child be like?
- How would my child affect my home?
- Am I physically and emotionally strong enough to care for my child?
- How will others treat me and my child?
- Could my family grow stronger in faith, love, and courage if I parent my baby?
- Will I be able to give time and love to my other children if I care for this child?
- Will I have time for myself?
- Can I emotionally handle a child with a terminal illness? How will I feel as my child's health declines?
- Will I be able to fully love my dying child? Or will I distance myself emotionally so as not to feel the loss?

Educational Considerations

- What educational opportunities are available for my child?
- Is early childhood stimulation possible?
- What type of education might help my child the most? Do local agencies or schools provide this?
- Are any books available so that I (or others) can learn the techniques?
- Will my child need tutoring at home? Does the local school system provide this?

Finding Help

- Who can provide practical help if I parent my child?
- Will someone else be able to parent for a while, so I can have time alone?
- Can I hire some part-time help such as teenaged baby sitters or others?
- Do I prefer to have a live-in housekeeper or baby sitter? Can I offer room, board, and a small salary to a live-in helper?
- Would youth groups, religious groups, or community service organizations provide some free daily or weekly care for my child in order to give me a break?
- Does my city have a facility that would take my child days? How about overnight or for a weekend occasionally?
- Can another mother and I occasionally take turns child sitting?
- Can someone help with grocery shopping, child care, or stimulation exercises for my child?
- Is respite care available in my area? What does it cost?
- If I have a low income or receive public assistance, might my caseworker or social worker be able to arrange for some homemaker assistance for me?
- Will I have to lobby for help for my child?

A Plan for the Child Who Has Special Needs or a Terminal Illness

Each child is unique, as is each mother and each family. What may work for another mother or another family may not work for yours. Be honest about your abilities and desires. Choose a plan that will be best for you and for your child.

CREATING AN ADOPTION PLAN

If adoption is a good choice, you can choose the type of plan you want. First, answer these questions alone. Then review them with a few adoption counselors. If you know what type of plan you want, you can choose a consultant who can help you make that plan.

Involving Others

- Would I want to have my pregnancy public knowledge or do I prefer to keep things quiet?
- Do I want to put this whole experience behind me?
- Would I want my husband to know about my pregnancy? If I'm not married, would I want to tell my future husband about my baby?
- How will my husband react if I keep in contact with my child? Would he feel threatened? If he did, could I choose between my husband and my child?
- If I now have or ever have had other children, how will they feel about adoption?
- Will it be good for my other children to know how their brother or sister is doing?
- Which type of arrangement could my other children best deal with?
- How will keeping in touch with my child affect my future? How about having no contact?

Knowledge of Your Child's Progress

- Would I want to know where my child is and how my child is doing?
- Would I want to choose and meet my child's adoptive family?
- Would I ever want to see my child again?
- Do I want to assume any responsibility for my child? How much?
- What will I feel if I know my child's whereabouts? Will knowing cause me emotional strain?
- How will my child handle knowing who I am and where I am? How will the adoptive family feel?

Contact With Your Child

- What degree of involvement do I want with my child?
- Am I content to have no contact with my child after the adoption is complete?
- Would one or two yearly exchanges of information be enough for me?
- Would I want to visit my child? How often?
- Would my contact disturb the relationship my child has with the adoptive family? Would the child be "mine" or "theirs"? Could the child be "ours"? How do I feel about this? What is best for my child?
- Will the adoptive couple feel threatened if I know where my child is? If I write to my child? Visit?

Taking Your Child Into Consideration

- How will my child handle a relationship with me? How will this affect the relationship with the adoptive parents?
- How might my relationship with my child affect my child's sense of family, stability, and belonging?
- Can I be a biological mother and still allow my child to have a family other than my own?
- Will my presence have a good or bad effect on my child's self-image? Will my presence help my child or be confusing?
- Will my presence have any effect on my child's relationships with others, especially if I live nearby?
- How will I handle the following questions from my child: "Are you my real mommy?" "Why did you give me up?" "How could you give me up if you loved me?" "Do I have to listen to my adoptive family?" "Can I go home with you?"
- Would my child or I ever achieve the freedom necessary to go on with our own lives? Would we always have confusion and unresolved feelings in our relationship?
- What kind of relationship would I have with my child?
- Could I talk openly to my child about any problems I might be experiencing? Could my child talk to me?

Parenting Differences

- Would I want to parent my child? Would parenting be wise for me? Good for my child? What conflicts can I foresee with the adoptive family?
- Can I accept visiting my child without parenting my child?
- What if I don't like the way my child is being raised? Would I interfere?
- Is it good for my child to have two sets of parents and two sets of "rules"? If not, could I accept the parenting techniques of the adoptive family while keeping my own ideas to myself?

- Would I want to talk over some of my ideas with the adoptive family? What if the adoptive parents reject my ideas?
- Will careful choosing of the adoptive family enable me to find a family whose parenting style is similar to my own?

Emotional Conflicts

- If my situation improved, would I try to reclaim my child?
- What if my child doesn't meet my expectations? How will I react? How will I view the adoptive family? Will I blame them? Why or why not?
- How will I feel about conflicts between my child and the adoptive family? Whose side will I take?
- What if my child loves the adoptive family more than me? Would I try to "steal" my child's love?
- What if my child rejects the adoptive family in favor of me?
- Suppose my child wants to come home and live with me? What will I do? Can I rationally evaluate such a situation to determine if my child has valid reasons for wanting to leave the adoptive family? If my child is simply being rebellious or manipulative, what will I do?
- Suppose my child has valid reasons for wanting to reject the adoptive family. What will I do then? Who can help me make a wise decision in this case?

Living Near Your Child

- Would I want to live near the adoptive family or far from them? How would I handle either situation?
- Suppose the adoptive family moved away? Or moved nearby? Could I handle the new arrangement?
- Suppose I had to move away from or closer to my child? How would I feel about that?

Handling the Biological Father

- How will my child's biological father fit into the picture? Would I want him to know my child's whereabouts and be involved with my child?
- How will the adoptive family feel about the biological father?
- How will he answer the questions in this Appendix?
- Are the biological father and I in conflict over any of the answers to these questions? Can we resolve our conflicts?
- How will my ongoing relationship (if there is one) with my baby's father affect the adoption?
- What if he and I no longer get along, yet we still maintain contact with our child? Can we handle this situation?
- Suppose we should marry each other? How will we handle the adoptive situation?
- How will we handle each other's future spouses? What will be their relationships to our adopted child?

Finalizing an Adoption Plan

You have much to consider in making an adoption plan. You must consider your own needs and desires as well as those of the biological father and adoptive family. In addition, you must try to foresee how your child might respond to the plan you choose.

Don't just think about your plan. Talk it over with those you trust and those who have been involved in adoptions. You might even talk to some teens or adults who have been adopted. What type of plan would they choose for themselves?

Your answers to these questions, as well as the input of others, may cause you to change your plans a bit. Always try to choose what is best for all concerned, right now and in the long run.

CHOOSING AN ADOPTION CONSULTANT

Answering the questions earlier in this Appendix should help you determine what sort of adoption plan you want. Write down this plan. To find an adoption consultant who will help you make this plan, ask a few consultants the questions that follow. Write down the answers or tape-record them, then review them a few times before choosing a consultant to work with.

Questions About Plans the Consultant Offers

- What type of adoption plans do you offer? Will I be able to make the adoption plan I have chosen?
- Can you help to make an alternate parenting plan such as foster care, institutional care, or parenting by a relative?
- How much counseling will I receive? If I feel that I need more counseling, will I receive it? Suppose I feel that I need less counseling?
- What financial arrangements can you make for my health care? For other expenses?
- If I decide to parent my child myself, what bills will be my responsibility?
- What legal services do you offer? Who pays my legal fees?
- Will I be pressured to choose any option? Can I request another consultant at any time? Switch agencies? Make an alternative adoption plan?
- How will you handle my child's father? My desire for privacy? My family? Will I have to tell them about this adoption? Who else will I have to tell? What if I don't want to tell them?

Questions About the Consultant's Credentials

- Is this agency government sponsored? How does this affect me? How does it affect the adoptive family?
- Are you registered with a local business bureau? What references can this bureau give me about your firm? (You can check with the bureau on these.)
- What governmental office, such as a department for children and their families, would have information about you? What information can this office give me? (Again, check up on the consultant.)
- What can a legal association tell me about you as an adoption attorney or about the attorneys whom your agency consults?
- Do you provide references of clients previously served? May I speak to these references?
- How many adoptions have you arranged?
- How many adoptions do you plan to arrange this year?
- Can you arrange adoptions across state or national boundaries?
- How do you "find" birth mothers and adoptive families? Through advertising? Referral from doctors? Community agencies?
- What professional degrees do you hold?
- Are you a professional counselor? Lawyer? Psychologist?
- What type of adoption arrangement can you legally offer in this area? Can you refer me to someone else if this is not the plan I want?
- Who do you represent—me or the adoptive parents? If not me, alone, can you refer me to someone who will represent me?

Questions About the Consultant's Arrangements for the Baby

- How long will my baby have to wait to be adopted?
- Will my baby go into foster care before going to the adoptive family?
- How many adoptive families are you working with?
- If my baby has special needs or a terminal illness, can you place my baby with a family?
- How many families are willing to adopt children like mine?
- What counseling do adoptive parents receive?
- How are adoptive families chosen? What requirements must they meet?
- How carefully are adoptive families screened? Are any rejected? For what reasons?
- Can I choose my child's adoptive family? How?
- Can I choose my child's religious upbringing? Ethnic family background? Social status? Environment? Financial situation? Family makeup?
- Do you allow adoption by single parents?
- What happens to my child if the adoptive family divorces or one or both parents die? If my child is abused or neglected? Who checks on this?
- What type of parenting advice and instruction do you provide to adoptive parents?
- How do you check on the adoptive family after my child goes into their home?
- How can I be sure that these parents are the ones I want for my child?
- Can you arrange an adoption with a family that I know who wants to adopt my baby?

A Consultant Who Will Work for You

Interview several adoption consultants until you find one who will give you the type of plan you want. Then ask yourself if you feel comfortable talking to this person. Does this consultant respect your feelings and treat you as a person of worth, dignity, and intelligence? It's very important that you choose a consultant with whom you feel comfortable and whom you trust. Adoption can be an emotionally difficult choice even though it is the best choice for you and your baby. The right adoption consultant will guide you through the decision and provide answers and support.

Appendix H

USING SPECIAL AGENCIES

Agencies can provide much help. National headquarters can make local referrals. All 800 phone numbers are toll free. If a number is not an 800 number, you will have to pay for the call. Know in advance what information you need from the agency. Try to keep your calls short to minimize expenses. Or have a local PREGNANCY AIDgency call for you. Refer to the PREGNANCY AIDgency section of this Appendix.

If you reach an answering machine, try calling again. Or leave a brief message, your name, and your phone number, and offer to have the group call you back collect. Only a few agencies accept collect phone calls. A telephone operator can explain how to call collect, what code or number you must dial before dialing long distance, and if there is a time difference in the area you're calling. Some agencies are open twenty-four hours; others are open days or evenings only. The agencies here are just a sampling of the many available in the United States. PREGNANCY AIDgencies are listed worldwide.

A few of the groups listed in this Appendix have addresses only. When writing to a group, always enclose a self-addressed, stamped, business-size (4 inch by 9 inch) envelope for a reply. If you are writing to a group in another country, speak to a post office official regarding the type and amount of postage to include with your return envelope.

The information in this Appendix is current as of May 1990. Please notify the author, through the publisher, of any changes, additions, and deletions, and whether agencies were helpful or not so helpful, for use in revising this section.

The agencies, organizations, groups, and others listed in this Appendix can provide much help, referral, or advice. Mention of these agencies, organizations, groups, and others in this Appendix does not imply that they adhere to any specific philosophy regarding abortion.

COMMUNITY RESOURCES

With a PREGNANCY AIDgency or other group, approach the following community agencies for financial aid, volunteer assistance, and donations of food, clothes, and other necessities.

- Churches, synagogues
- Councils of churches
- Prominent individuals, business people
- Businesses, corporations
- Campaign for Human Development, Lutheran Social Services, other fund drives
- Civic organizations, service clubs
- Knights of Columbus, Masons, Elks, Rotary, Lions, Business and Professional Women, JayCees, Junior Optimist, Junior League, Kiwanis, etc.
- Religious organizations, prayer groups
- Chamber of Commerce
- Youth groups, civic and religious
- Newspaper (for publicity)
- Self-help groups
- United Way

To locate community groups, refer to your telephone book or newspaper, or seek help from your friends, the town hall, or local bodies of worship.

ENCYCLOPEDIA OF ASSOCIATIONS

The *Encyclopedia of Associations*, published in the United States by Gale Research Company, describes thousands of national groups, listing addresses, phone numbers, contacts, and services. Other countries have similar references. Most libraries have these books. If yours doesn't, call a library in a large city and ask the librarian to locate, in this reference, the groups dealing with your problem and to give you the phone numbers. National organizations can provide information and referrals.

GOVERNMENT AGENCIES

Call your town hall for referral to government agencies offering assistance to needy women and their children. A PREGNANCY AIDgency can act as an advocate for you.

HOTLINE DIRECTORY

A directory of toll-free, help agency hotlines is available in the United States for one dollar. Write to *Hotline Guide*, Essential Information, P.O. Box 19405, Washington, DC 20036, and enclose a self-addressed, stamped, business-size (4 inch by 9 inch) envelope, or phone 202/387-8030. These hotlines provide much information and referral on a variety of topics. The directory is an excellent resource.

If you have trouble reaching an 800 number, call toll-free directory assistance at 800/555-1212 for help.

PREGNANCY AIDGENCIES

As discussed in Chapter Two, "PREGNANCY AIDgency" is a term coined for use in this book. It refers to the thousands of pregnancy help agencies that exist worldwide under a variety of names. To locate a local agency to help you, or to find a complete listing of PREGNANCY AIDgencies under their various names, call the numbers below. They can refer you.

Most PREGNANCY AIDgencies accept collect phone calls if you are unable to pay. However, remember that these agencies have limited funds. Paying for your call, if you are able to do so, is very helpful.

International Referral

☐ **Alternatives to Abortion, International**
c/o Margaret Hartshorn, Ph.D., and the Women's Health and Educational Foundation
1213½ South James Road
Columbus, Ohio 43227
614/239-WHEF
614/444-4411

Distributes a directory of PREGNANCY AIDgencies worldwide. Referral to Australia, Austria, Belgium, Canada, Columbia, Cyprus, France, Germany, Gibraltar, Holland, India, Ireland, Italy, Japan, Netherlands, New Zealand, Norway, Poland, Puerto Rico, Scotland, South Africa, Spain, Sweden, Taiwan, United Kingdom, United States, Uruguay, Venezuela, West Africa, and Yugoslavia. If you don't live in one of these countries, visit an agency in a nearby country.

☐ **Human Life International**
Gaithersburg, Maryland
301/670-7884

Human Life International does not list specific PREGNANCY AIDgencies worldwide, but it does have pro-life contacts in many countries. Call Human Life International to locate these contacts. Contact persons will probably be able to refer you to PREGNANCY AIDgencies. Human Life International does not accept collect phone calls since it is an information group, not a PREGNANCY AIDgency.

United States PREGNANCY AIDgency Referral Lines

☐ **AAO (Alpha and Omega) Problem Pregnancy Helpline**
800/228-0332

☐ **Bethany Christian Services**
800/BETHANY

☐ **Birthright, USA**
800/848-LOVE

☐ **Christian Action Council**
Falls Church, Virginia
703/237-2100

☐ **Georgia Nurses for Life**
Atlanta, Georgia
404/447-1598

Possible referral to medical professionals, nationwide. Does not accept collect phone calls.

☐ **International Life Services**
Los Angeles, California
213/382-2156

☐ **Lifeline Crisis Pregnancy Hotline**
800/852-LOVE

☐ **Nurturing Network**
Boise, Idaho
208/344-7200

Emphasis on college and career women.

☐ **Pearson Foundation**
St. Louis, Missouri
800/633-2252, Ext. 700
314/772-2228

☐ **Pregnancy Counseling Service Liberty Godparent Foundation**
800/368-3336

☐ **Several Sources Foundation**
Ramsey, New Jersey
201/825-7277

Mother and children's shelter and other services.

Other English-Speaking Countries PREGNANCY AIDgency Referral

Australia

☐ **APPC (Action Pregnancy Problem Centre) in Victoria**
—03/783-6250 (Frankston)
—052/22-1453 (Geelong)
—051/34-7254 (Morwell)
—055/62-6679 (Warrnambool)
—058/21-0991 (Shepparton)
—054/415-795 (Bendigo)

☐ **Birthline**
Hackney, South Australia
08/363-1444

☐ **Caroline Chisholm Society**
Moonee Ponds, Victoria
03/370-3933

☐ **Pregnancy Action Centre**
Ringwood, Victoria
03/870-7044

British Isles (England, Ireland, Scotland, Wales)

☐ **LIFE**
Warwickshire, England
0926-421587
0926-311511

Canada

☐ **Alliance for Life**
Winnipeg, Manitoba
800/665-0570
204/942-4772

☐ **Beginnings**
Hamilton, Ontario
416/528-6665

☐ **Birthright, Canada**
Toronto, Canada
800/328-LOVE
416/469-1111

☐ **Catholic Foundation for Human Life**
Moncton, New Brunswick
506/858-1011

☐ **Crisis Pregnancy Centre**
Calgary, Alberta
403/245-9000

☐ **Respect Life Centre**
Antigonish, Nova Scotia
902/863-6636

Tasmania

☐ **Tasmania Pregnancy Support Services**
Hobart, Tasmania
02/34-7561

New Zealand

☐ **Pregnancy Counseling**
Auckland, New Zealand
09/521-4125

☐ **Pregnancy Help**
Auckland, New Zealand
09/732-599

PRO-LIFE DENOMINATIONAL GROUPS

Pro-life denominational groups *may* refer you to bodies of worship or individuals who can provide some help. Most of these cannot afford to accept collect phone calls.

☐ **Catholics United for Life**
New Hope, Kentucky
502/325-3061

☐ **Christians for Life**
Oshawa, Ontario
416/434-7977

☐ **Christian Life Commission of the Southern Baptist Convention**
Nashville, Tennessee
615/244-2495

☐ **Jewish Anti-Abortion League**
c/o Rabbi Yehuda Levin
P.O. Box 262 Grazesend Station
Brooklyn, New York 11223

☐ **Lutherans for Life**
Minneapolis, Minnesota
612/721-3037

☐ **Methodists for Life**
Steve Wissler
Ephrata, Pennsylvania
717/738-2724

☐ **Moravians for Life**
Lake Mills, Wisconsin
414/648-2402

☐ **National Conference of Catholic Bishops**
Washington, DC
202/541-3000

☐ **National Organization of Episcopalians for Life**
Fairfax, Virginia
703/591-6635

☐ **Presbyterians for Life**
Minneapolis, Minnesota
612/861-5346

☐ **United Church of Christ Friends for Life**
Reverend John Brown
Bechtelsville, Pennsylvania
215/754-6446

SELF-HELP GROUPS

Self-help groups help their members deal with specific problems. PREGNANCY AIDgencies, religious institutions, government agencies, hospitals, newspapers, phone books, and telephone operator assistance may list self-help groups. Or call one of the following:

☐ **The National Self-Help Clearing House**
New York, New York
212/642-2944

☐ **The New Jersey Self-Help Clearing House**
St. Clare's-Riverside Medical Center
Pocono Road
Denville, New Jersey 07834
201/625-9565
201/625-7101

Distributes *The Self-Help Sourcebook: Finding and Forming Mutual Aid Self-Help Groups.* Reasonably priced. Lists over 1,000 United States self-help groups. Information on forming self-help groups.

To prevent overlapping of information, this Appendix of *Having Your Baby When Others Say No!* does *not* list groups found in *The Self-Help Sourcebook. Sourcebook* groups deal with the following problems:

• Adoption, foster care
• Aging
• Caretakers of ill, aged
• Childbirth, Cesarean birth
• Addictions (eating disorders, overweight, drugs, alcoholism, sex gambling, smoking)
• Physical disabilities

- Mental disabilities, mental illness retardation
- Disease, accident victims
- Battering, child abuse
- Sexual trauma
- Parenting groups
- Special needs and terminally ill children
- Crime victims, offenders
- Death of spouse, child, or self, miscarriage, infertility
- Debt
- Marriage, divorce, single parenthood, separation
- Learning disabilities
- Rare disorders, genetic disorders

☐ **Self-Help Center**
Evanston, Illinois
708/328-0470

SPECIFIC AGENCIES

These agencies are a few of the thousands available. National self-help clearing houses, PREGNANCY AIDgencies, government offices, hospitals, professionals, and the *Encyclopedia of Associations* can refer you to many additional groups.

ABUSE AND ASSAULT

☐ **Boys Town National Hotline**
800/448-3000

All ages referral to safety.

☐ **Childhelp National Child Abuse Hotline**
800/4-A-CHILD

☐ **CONTACT: Parents United International and Institute for the Community as Extended Family**
Peggy Stoddard
San Jose, California
408/453-7611, Ext. 150

Youth and adult incest victims.

☐ **Domestic Violence Project Learning Center Inc.**
Paul and Judy Hegstrom
Quincy, Illinois
217/222-3711

Treatment program for violent men and their wives.

☐ **INTAKE**
San Jose, California
408/453-0727

Victims of incest.

☐ **Life After Assault League**
Kay Zibolsky
Appleton, Wisconsin
414/739-4489

Christian counseling for rape and incest victims.

☐ **National Council on Child Abuse and Family Violence**
800/222-2000

☐ **National Domestic Violence Hotline**
800/333-SAFE

Referral to local shelters for battered women.

☐ **Parents Anonymous**
800/421-0353
Child abuse.

ADDICTIONS

☐ **Alcohol and Drug Referral Helpline**
800-ALCOHOL

24-hour hotline.

☐ **Intergroup Association of Alcoholics Anonymous of New York**
New York, New York
212/683-3900

☐ **Kids Are Special**
San Jose, California
408/297-5437

Children living in alcoholic families.

☐ **National Association for Children of Alcoholics**
South Laguna, California
714/499-3889

☐ **National Institute on Drug Abuse Hotline**
800/662-HELP

☐ **New Hope for Adult Children of Alcoholics**
Fullerton, California
714/529-5544

Evangelical church.

☐ **Self-Injury Hotline**
800/DONT CUT

☐ **Stop Smoking Program**
c/o American Cancer Society
Atlanta, Georgia
404/892-0026

☐ **Substance Abuse Hotline**
800/992-9239

ADOPTION

☐ **Adoption Center**
800/448-KIDS

☐ **American Adoption Congress**
New York, New York
212/988-0110

☐ **Bethany Christian Services**
800/BETHANY

☐ **Birthmother Hotline**
800/392-2121

☐ **Chosen Children**
Louisville, Kentucky
502/491-6410

☐ **Council of Three Rivers American Indian Center, Inc.**
Pittsburgh, Pennsylvania
412/782-4457

Native American adoption.

☐ **Golden Cradle**
Cherry Hill, New Jersey
609/667-2229

☐ **International Soundex Reunion Registry**
Carson City, Nevada
702/882-7755

Mutual consent reunion registry for birth parents, children, adult siblings. Medic alert, genetic outreach.

☐ **Liberty Godparent Foundation Pregnancy Counseling Service**
800/368-3336

☐ **National Adoption Center**
800/TO-ADOPT

☐ **National Adoption Exchange**
Philadelphia, Pennsylvania
215/925-0200

Adoption of special needs children, siblings.

☐ **New Beginning Consulting Service, Inc.**
Santa Ana, California
714/973-4569

☐ **Rootwings Ministries**
Barre, Vermont
802/479-2197
413/586-5682

Adoption of children with special needs or terminal illnesses.

☐ **Up With Down Syndrome Foundation**
Miami, Florida
305/386-9115

Adoption of Down Syndrome children.

☐ **World Adoption International Fund (WAIF)**
New York, New York
212/533-2558

EATING DISORDERS

☐ **American Anorexia/Bulimia Association, Inc.**
New York, New York
212/734-1114

☐ **The Connection/Weight Watchers International**
800/333-3000

☐ **National Eating Disorder Hotline**
Baltimore, Maryland
301/332-9800

☐ **TOPS (Take Off Pounds Sensibly) Club**
Milwaukee, Wisconsin
414/482-4620

☐ **3D (Diet, Discipline, Discipleship)
Diet Plan**
800/451-5006

Diet plan, counseling.

EDUCATION AND CAREER ASSISTANCE

☐ **Business and Professional Women's
Foundation**
Washington, DC
202/293-1200

☐ **Center for Family Business**
Mayfield Heights, Ohio
216/442-0800

☐ **HEATH Resource Center**
800/54-HEATH

Information about educational opportunities for adults with disabilities.

☐ **Homeworkers Organized for More
Employment**
Orland, Maine
207/469-7961

Sale of homemade crafts.

☐ **Human Resources Development
Institute**
Washington, DC
202/638-3912

Dislocated and economically disadvantaged workers.

☐ **Job Accommodation Network**
800/526-7234

Modifications in the workplace for persons with disabilities.

☐ **Learning Resources Network**
Manhattan, Kansas
913/539-5376

☐ **National Center for American Indian
Enterprise Development**
El Monte, California
818/442-3701

☐ **National Congress of Neighborhood
Women**
Brooklyn, New York
718/388-6666

Working class women.

☐ **National Literacy Hotline**
800/228-8813

☐ **National Women's Employment
and Education**
Los Angeles, California
213/489-7117

☐ **Small Business Administration**
800/368-5855

☐ **Student Financial Aid**
800/333-4636

☐ **Vocational Education**
800/443-1771

☐ **Women's American ORT
(Organization for Rehabilitation
Through Training)**
New York, New York
212/505-7700

Vocational education and training.

☐ **Women's Sports Foundation**
800/227-3988

EMOTIONAL PEACE

☐ **Anxiety Disorders Association
of America (ADAA)**
Rockville, Maryland
301/231-9350

☐ **Christian Association
for Psychological Studies**
P.O. Box 628
Blue Jay, California 92319

Referral to local Christian psychologists and psychiatrists. However, check to be sure that any psychologist is supportive of your desire to give birth to your baby.

☐ **Minirth-Meier Clinic**
800/232-9462

☐ **National Mental Health Association**
Alexandria, Virginia
703/684-7722

☐ **Recovery**
Chicago, Illinois
312/337-5661

Self-help for mental patients.

FAMILY PLANNING AND BIRTH CONTROL

☐ **American Academy of Natural Family Planning**
St. Louis, Missouri
314/569-6495

☐ **Association for Voluntary Surgical Contraception**
New York, New York
212/351-2500

☐ **Birth Control Care Center**
800/255-7889

☐ **Couple to Couple League**
Cincinnati, Ohio
513/661-7612

Natural family planning.

FINANCES

☐ **Debtors Anonymous General Service Board**
P.O. Box 20322
New York, New York 10025-9992

HEALTH AND SPECIAL NEEDS INFORMATION

Thousands of organizations deal with health problems and special needs concerns. Get the latest information before making any decisions.

☐ **Accent on Information**
Bloomington, Illinois
309/378-2961

☐ **Accreditation of Rehabilitation Facilities**
Tucson, Arizona
602/748-1212

Accredits organizations that provide services to persons with disabilities.

☐ **Council for Exceptional Children**
Reston, Virginia
703/620-3660

Education.

☐ **Direct Link**
Solvang, California
805/688-1603

Information, referral, case advocacy for persons with disabilities.

☐ **East Coast Migrant Health Project**
Washington, DC
202/347-7377

☐ **Exceptional Parent Bookstore and Magazine**
Boston, Massachusetts
617/730-5800

☐ **Foundation for Exceptional Children**
Reston, Virginia
703/620-1054

☐ **Information Center for General Health Problems**
800/221-5517

☐ **Information Center for Individuals With Disabilities**
Boston, Massachusetts
617/727-5540

☐ **Medicare Special Issues and Second Surgical Opinions**
800/638-6833
In Maryland 800/492-6603

Second opinion referrals for surgery and treatment.

☐ **National Center for Education in Maternal and Child Health**
Washington, DC
202/625-8400
202/625-8410

☐ **National Information Center for Children and Youth With Handicaps**
800/999-5599

☐ **National Information System and Clearinghouse for Health Related Services**
800/922-9234

☐ **National Organization for Rare Disorders (NORD)**
New Fairfield, Connecticut
800/447-6673
203/746-6518

☐ **National Organization on Disability**
800/248-ABLE

☐ **National Rehabilitation Information Center**
800/34-NARIC

☐ **National Support Center for Persons With Disabilities**
800/426-2133

Technology and other referral.

☐ **ODPHP (Office of Disease Prevention and Health Promotion) National Health Information Center**
800/336-4797

☐ **Parent Information Center**
Concord, New Hampshire
603/224-7005

☐ **Pediatricians for Life**
Dr. Eugene F. Diamond
Chicago, Illinois
312/233-8000

Specific Health Concerns

These are a few of the many groups providing information on specific health and special needs topics.

☐ **AIDS National Hotline**
800/342-2437 (English)
800/344-7432 (Spanish)
800/243-7889 (for the hearing impaired)

☐ **AMC Cancer Research Center**
800/525-3777

☐ **American Academy of Allergy and Immunology**
Milwaukee, Wisconsin
414/272-6071

☐ **American Council of Blind Parents**
800/424-8666

☐ **American Diabetes Association**
800/232-3472
In Virginia and Washington, DC
703/549-1500

☐ **American Foundation for the Blind**
800/AF-BLIND

☐ **American Kidney Fund**
800/638-8299
In Maryland 800/492-8361

Kidney disease.

☐ **American Society for Dermatologic Surgery**
800/441-ASDS

Surgery for genital warts.

☐ **American Speech-Language-Hearing Association**
800/638-8255
In Maryland 301/897-8682

☐ **Association for Retarded Citizens**
Arlington, Texas
817/640-0204

☐ **Autism Society of America**
Washington, DC
202/783-0125

☐ **Better Hearing Institute**
800/424-8576
In Virginia 703/642-0580

☐ **Billy Barty Foundation for Little People**
4007 West Magnolia Boulevard
Burbank, California 91505-2824

For anyone 4′10″ or under.

☐ **Cancer Care, Inc.**
New York, New York
212/221-3300

Care to cancer victims and families.

☐ **Cancer Response Service**
800/227-2345

☐ **Cansurmount**
Atlanta, Georgia
404/320-3333

Cancer victims helping other cancer patients and their families.

☐ **Center for Sickle Cell Disease**
Washington, DC
202/636-7930

☐ **Children in Hospitals**
Boston, Massachusetts
617/482-2915
Needham, Massachusetts
617/444-3877

☐ **Family Community Resources**
Rockville, Maryland
301/984-5792

Support group and advocate for Down Syndrome children in the community and school. Provides respite care and has an extensive library.

☐ **Foundation for Hospice and Homecaring**
Washington, DC
202/547-6586

☐ **Health and Light Foundation**
800/LIGHTS-U

Effect of natural and artificial lighting on health.

☐ **Hope for the Handicapped**
Budd Lake, New Jersey
201/691-1836

Gospel on tape.

☐ **International Center for Artificial Organs and Transplantation**
Cleveland, Ohio
216/421-0757

☐ **International Craniofacial Foundation**
800/535-3643

☐ **Joni & Friends**
Agoura, California
818/707-5664

Children with special needs or health problems.

☐ **Little People of America**
Washington, DC
301/589-0730

Dwarfism.

☐ **Malta Center**
Phoenix, Arizona
602/230-1881

Spiritual counseling for AIDS patients.

☐ **March of Dimes Birth Defects Foundation**
National Headquarters
White Plains, New York
914/428-7100

☐ **Medicare**
800/462-9306

☐ **Michael Fund International Foundation for Genetic Research**
Monroeville, Pennsylvania
412/823-6380

☐ **Muscular Dystrophy Association**
New York, New York
212/586-0808

☐ **National Asthma Center/Jewish Lung Line**
800/222-LUNG

☐ **National Cancer Institute**
800/4-CANCER

☐ **National Center for Stuttering**
800/221-2483

☐ **National Down Syndrome Society**
800/221-4602

☐ **National Easter Seal Society, Inc.**
Chicago, Illinois
312/726-6200

Helps persons with activity limitations achieve maximum independence.

☐ **National Industries for the Severely Handicapped**
Vienna, Virginia
703/560-6800

☐ **National Lupus Erythematosus Foundation (NLEF)**
North Ridge, California
818/885-8787

☐ **National Parkinson Foundation**
800/327-4545

☐ **National Spinal Cord Injury Association**
Woburn, Massachusetts
617/935-2722

☐ **National STD (Sexually Transmitted Disease) Hotline**
800/227-8922

☐ **Orton Dyslexia Society**
800/ABCD-123

☐ **Pesticide Information**
800/858-7378

☐ **Pilot Parents**
Omaha, Nebraska
402/346-5220

Support groups for parents of children with special needs.

☐ **PMS Access**
800/222-4-PMS

Premenstrual syndrome.

☐ **Project Concern**
San Diego, California
619/279-9690

Health care for rural America and around the world.

☐ **RESNA**
Washington, DC
202/857-1199

Technology for persons with disabilities.

☐ **Retarded Infants Services**
New York, New York
212/889-5464

☐ **Safe Drinking Water**
800/426-4791

☐ **Shriners Hospitals for Crippled Children**
800/237-5055
In Florida 800/282-9161

☐ **Spina Bifida Association of America**
800/621-3141

☐ **TASH: The Association for Persons With Severe Handicaps**
Seattle, Washington
206/523-8446

☐ **Teen TAP**
800/234-TEEN

AIDS information for teens.

☐ **United Cerebral Palsy Association**
800/USA-1UCP

☐ **World Federation of Doctors Who Respect Human Life**
Oak Park, Illinois
708/383-8766

☐ **Young Adult Institute and Workshop**
New York, New York
212/563-7474

Respite services for homes with special needs or ill children.

HOMES AND SCHOOLS FOR CHILDREN WITH SPECIAL NEEDS OR HEALTH PROBLEMS

The following are some of the many excellent institutions, schools, and group homes for children with special needs or health problems.

☐ **The Hope School**
Springfield, Illinois
217/786-3350

Blind children with other disabilities.

☐ **Misericordia Heart of Mercy Center**
Chicago, Illinois
312/254-9595
312/973-6300

☐ **National Benevolent Association (NBA) of the Christian Church (Disciples of Christ)**
St. Louis, Missouri
314/993-9000

Referral.

☐ **Our Lady of Victory Infant Home**
Lackawanna, New York
716/827-9611

☐ **St. John's Children's Home/St. John of God Community Services**
Carrollton, Ohio
216/627-7647

☐ **School for Special Children**
Westville Grove, New Jersey
609/848-4700

☐ **Seven Sorrows of Our Sorrowful Mother Infants' Home, Inc.**
Necedah, Wisconsin
608/565-2417

LEGAL HELP

☐ **American Bar Association**
800/621-6159
In Illinois 312/988-5000

☐ **Attorney Referral Network**
800/624-8846

☐ **Migrant Legal Action Program**
Washington, DC
202/462-7744

☐ **National Association of Protection and Advocacy Systems**
Washington, DC
202/546-8202

Legal aid for persons with disabilities.

☐ **The Rutherford Institute**
c/o John W. Whitehead
P.O. Box 7482
Charlottesville, Virginia 22906-7482

MARRIAGE PREPARATION AND ENRICHMENT

☐ **Ackerman Institute for Family Therapy**
New York, New York
212/879-4900

☐ **American Association for Marriage and Family**
Washington, DC
202/429-1825

☐ **Christian Marriage Enhancement**
Temple, Texas
817/771-5571

☐ **Christian Marriage Enrichment**
Tustin, California
714/544-7560

☐ **International Marriage Encounter**
St. Paul, Minnesota
612/454-6434

☐ **Interracial Family Alliance**
Houston, Texas
713/454-5018

☐ **World Wide Marriage Encounter**
San Bernardino, California
714/881-3456

MATERNITY HOMES

Maternity homes are group homes for women in pregnancy crisis. A local PREGNANCY AIDgency can refer you to maternity homes in your area. Some representative homes are presented in the following list.

☐ **Bethany Maternity Home**
800/BETHANY

☐ **Chosen Children Maternity Home**
Louisville, Kentucky
502/491-6410

☐ **Edna Gladney Maternity Home**
800/433-2922

☐ **Liberty Godparent Home**
800/368-3336

☐ **The Mary Weslin Home, Inc.**
Colorado Springs, Colorado
719/390-8584

☐ **St. Anne's Maternity Home**
Los Angeles, California
213/381-2931

☐ **Seven Sorrows of Our Sorrowful Mother Infants' Home, Inc.**
Necedah, Wisconsin
608/565-2417

PARENTING AND FAMILY LIVING SKILLS

☐ **ASPO Lamaze, Inc.**
800/368-4404
In Virginia 703/524-7802

Referral to Lamaze childbirth classes.

☐ **Childbirth Hotline for the Bradley Method of Childbirth**
800/423-2397
In California 800/42-BIRTH

☐ **The Children's Foundation**
Washington, DC
202/347-3300

Children's food programs.

☐ **FEMALE (Formerly Employed Mothers at Loose Ends)**
P.O. Box 31
Elmhurst, Illinois 60126

Stay-at-home moms coping with small children.

☐ **Feminists for Life**
Kansas City, Missouri
816/753-2130

Feminists providing pregnancy support to other feminists.

☐ **Food Research and Action Center**
Washington, DC
202/393-5060

Federal food programs for the needy.

☐ **Home by Choice**
Box 103
Vienna, Virginia 22180

Career mothers who choose to stay at home with family.

☐ **HOPE Network for Single Mothers**
P.O. Box 232
Menomonee Falls, Wisconsin 53051

Write for information on starting a single mothers' support network.

☐ **International THEOS Foundation**
Pittsburgh, Pennsylvania
412/471-7779

Widows and widowers.

☐ **La Leche League International**
Franklin Park, Illinois
708/455-7730

Breastfeeding, early child rearing.

☐ **Messies Anonymous**
Miami, Florida
305/271-8404

Housekeeping organization.

☐ **Mothers at Home**
P.O. Box 2208
Merrifield, Virginia 22116

Publishes monthly newsletter for at-home moms.

☐ **Mothers of Pre-Schoolers (MOPS) International**
4175 Harlan Street, #105
Wheat Ridge, Colorado 80033

Group meetings for moms, babysitting for kids.

☐ **Mothers of Twins Clubs, Inc.**
Albuquerque, New Mexico
505/275-0955

☐ **National Academy of Nannies**
Denver, Colorado
303/333-NANI

☐ **National Child Support Advocacy Coalition**
P.O. Box 4629
Alexandria, Virginia 22306

☐ **Stepfamily Association of America**
Lincoln, Nebraska
402/477-7837

☐ **Super Women Anonymous**
San Francisco, California
415/928-3600

☐ **WARM**
San Jose, California
408/279-0303

Latch key children who are home alone for part of the day.

POST-ABORTION COUNSELING

☐ **American Rights Coalition**
800/634-2224

☐ **American Victims of Abortion**
Washington, DC
202/626-8800

☐ **Legal Action for Women**
Litigation Project
800/962-2319
In Florida 904/474-1091

☐ **National Office of Post Abortion**
Reconciliation and Healing
Milwaukee, Wisconsin
414/483-4141

☐ **Open ARMS**
Indianapolis, Indiana
317/359-9950

Abortion-related ministries for Christians.

☐ **PACE (Post Abortion Counseling**
and Education)
Tucson, Arizona
602/622-5774

☐ **Project Rachel**
Milwaukee, Wisconsin
414/769-3391

Sponsored by the Catholic Church.

☐ **Women Exploited by Abortion**
(WEBA) International
24823 Nogal
Moreno Valley, California 92388

PREGNANCY AND INFANT LOSS

These groups provide many resources and sometimes referral to local parent support groups.

☐ **Association for Recognizing**
the Life of Stillborns
Littleton, Colorado
303/978-9517

Will mail certificate of life to parents experiencing pregnancy loss.

☐ **National Center for the Prevention**
of Sudden Infant Death
Syndrome (SIDS)
800/638-7437

☐ **Nat'l SHARE**
Belleville, Illinois
618/234-2415

Referral to local support groups.

☐ **Our Newsletter**
Palmer, Alaska
907/745-2706

Loss of twin or other multiple birth child.

☐ **Pregnancy and Infant Loss Center**
Wayzata, Minnesota
612/473-9372

Reading materials, preborn burial cradles and burial gowns, newsletter, referral to local support groups.

☐ **Resolve Through Sharing (RTS)**
LaCrosse, Wisconsin
608/791-4747

Reading materials, local referral, counseling.

PRISONERS

Most of these agencies do not accept collect phone calls. Prisoners who cannot pay for calls should write.

☐ **AIM (Aid to Incarcerated Mothers)**
Jean Fox, Executive Director
Berkley Street, Fourth Floor
Suite 410
Boston, Massachusetts 02116
617/695-1588

☐ **Alston Wilkes Society**
2215 Devine Street
Columbia, South Carolina 29205
803/799-2490

Ex-offenders and their families.

☐ **Contact Center, Inc.**
Human Services Department
P.O. Box 81826
Lincoln, Nebraska 68501
402/464-0602

☐ **Friends Outside**
2105 Hamilton Avenue, Suite 290
San Jose, California 95125
408/879-0691

☐ **Legal Services for Prisoners
With Children**
1535 Mission Street
San Francisco, California 94103
415/552-3150

☐ **Prison Fellowship**
P.O. Box 17500
Washington, DC 20041-0500
703/478-0100
703/478-0452/FAX

☐ **Prison Ministries With Women**
P.O. Box 1911
Decatur, Georgia 30031-1911
404/622-4314

PROSTITUTION

These homes offer shelter, counsel, and concrete help in leaving prostitution.

☐ **Covenant House**
800/999-9999

☐ **Genesis House**
Chicago, Illinois
312/281-3917

SINGLE PARENT GROUP HOMES

These representative homes can help the single mother with shelter, parenting, and job skills.

☐ **Cardinal Cooke Residence**
Spring Valley, New York
914/356-0517

☐ **Covenant House**
800/999-9999

☐ **Good Counsel**
Staten Island, New York
718/727-8266

☐ **His Nesting Place**
Long Beach, California
213/422-2137

☐ **Hope House**
Savannah, Georgia
912/236-5310

☐ **Mom's House**
Johnstown, Pennsylvania
814/535-4848

☐ **Our Father's House**
Milton, Florida
904/626-9708

☐ **St. Francis Home**
Hoboken, New Jersey
201/798-9059

SPECIAL CIRCUMSTANCES

☐ **Association of Multi-Ethnic
Americans (AMEA)**
San Francisco, California
415/548-9300

☐ **Call for Action**
Washington, DC
202/686-8225

Consumer action.

☐ **Cult Crime Impact Network**
Boise, Idaho
208/377-6606

☐ **Enterprise Foundation**
Columbia, Maryland
301/964-1230

Low income housing and other needs.

☐ **Habitat for Humanity**
Americas, Georgia
912/924-6935

Low cost housing.

☐ **Housing Discrimination Hotline**
800/424-8590

☐ **National Cooperative Business
Association**
Washington, DC
202/638-6222

Helps form co-ops, including food co-ops.

☐ **Office for Civil Rights Hotline**
800/368-1019

Discrimination in hospitals, medical care.

☐ **Operation PUSH**
Chicago, Illinois
312/373-3366

Help for disadvantaged.

☐ **Warneke Ministries**
800/345-0045
In Kentucky 606/748-9961

Counseling for those formerly involved in the occult, Satanism, cults, or other controlling groups.

SUICIDE/RUNAWAYS

☐ **Boys Town National Hotline**
800/448-3000

☐ **Covenant House**
800/999-9999

☐ **National Runaway Switchboard and Suicide Hotline**
800/621-4000

☐ **Runaway Hotline**
800/231-6946
In Texas 800/392-3352

☐ **Samaritans**
Boston, Massachusetts
617/247-0220

TERMINAL ILLNESS

☐ **Children's Hospice International**
Alexandria, Virginia
703/684-0330

☐ **First Sunday**
Father Russ Kohler
Detroit, Michigan
313/832-4357

Terminally ill children and adults and their families.

☐ **Hospice**
Branford, Connecticut
203/481-6231

☐ **Hospicelink**
800/331-1620

☐ **St. Francis Center**
Washington, DC
202/363-8500

Support for those facing their own death or that of another.

TOTAL LIFE COUNSELING

The following groups offer much assistance in all aspects of life.

☐ **American Friends Service Committee**
Philadelphia, Pennsylvania
215/241-7000

☐ **Boys Town National Hotline**
800/448-3000

☐ **Community Transportation Association of America**
Washington, DC
202/628-1480

Transportation and other information services for needy rural people.

☐ **Covenant House**
800/999-9999

☐ **Humanistic Mental Health Foundation Hotline**
800/333-4444

Suicide, rape, drug abuse.

☐ **International Rescue Committee**
New York, New York
212/679-0010

Refugees.

☐ **KID NET**
800/543-6381

Teens.

☐ **Lutheran Immigration and Refugee Service**
New York, New York
212/532-6350

Immigrants and refugees.

☐ **National Coalition of Hispanic Health and Human Services Organizations**
Washington, DC
202/371-2100

☐ **National Indian Youth Council, Inc.**
Albuquerque, New Mexico
505/247-2251

☐ **National Urban League**
New York, New York
212/310-9000

Economically and socially disadvantaged.

☐ **National Youth Crisis Hotline**
800/HIT-HOME

Teens.

☐ **Salvation Army**
Verona, New Jersey
201/239-0606

☐ **United Native Americans**
Pinole, California
415/758-8160

Appendix I

READING FOR IDEAS

These books are representative of the thousands available in libraries and bookstores. As of July 1989, they are all in print. If you have difficulty obtaining a book, are dissatisfied with a book, or have found another book especially helpful, please notify the author, through the publisher. Your comments will be useful in planning revisions of this book.

The listing of these books does not imply that their authors or publishers adhere to any specific views regarding abortion.

ABUSE AND ASSAULT

Bass, Ellen and Laura Davis. *The Courage to Heal: A Guide for Women Survivors of Child Sexual Abuse.* New York: Harper & Row, 1988.

—— and Joan Torres. *Men Who Hate Women and the Women Who Love Them: When Loving Hurts and You Don't Know Why.* New York: Bantam, 1986.

Davidson, Terry. *Conjugal Crime: Understanding and Changing the Wife Beating Pattern.* New York: Hawthorn, 1978.

Gateley, Edwina. *I Hear a Seed Growing.* Trabuco Canyon, CA: Source Books, 1990. For prostitutes and those who counsel them.

Leman, Dr. Kevin. *The Pleasers: Women Who Can't Say No and the Men Who Control Them.* New York: Dell, 1987.

Miller, Kathy C. *Healing the Angry Heart: A Strategy for Confident Mothering.* Lynwood, WA: Aglow, 1984. Written by a mother who used to abuse her children.

NiCarthy, Ginny. *Getting Free: A Handbook for Women in Abusive Relationships*, rev. ed. Seattle, WA: Seal, 1986.

Walters, Candace. *Invisible Wounds: What Every Woman Should Know About Sexual Assault.* Portland, OR: Multnomah, 1988.

Zibolsky, Kay with Lynda Allison. *Healing Hidden Hurts—How You Can Live Again, After Assault.* Wilson, NC: Star, 1989. Christian.

ADDICTIONS

Al-Anon Family Group Headquarters, Inc. Staff. *Al-Anon's Twelve Steps and Twelve Traditions.* New York: Al-Anon, 1986.

——. *Alateen: Hope for Children of Alcoholics.* New York: Al-Anon, 1986.

Alcoholics Anonymous. *Twelve Steps and Twelve Traditions.* New York: Alcoholics Anonymous World Services, Inc., 1981.

Bill B. *Compulsive Overeater.* Minneapolis, MN: CompCare, 1981.

Carnes, Patrick, Ph.D. *Out of the Shadows: Understanding Sexual Addiction.* Minneapolis, MN: CompCare, 1983.

Cauwels, Janice M. *Bulimia: The Binge-Purge Compulsion.* Garden City, NY: Doubleday, 1983.

Christian, Shanon with Margaret Johnson. *The Very Private Matter of Anorexia Nervosa.* Grand Rapids, MI: Zondervan, 1986.

Fishel, Ruth. *Learning to Live in the Now: Six Week Personal Plan to Recovery.* Pompano Beach, FL: Health Communications, 1988. Recovery from addiction.

Hope and Recovery: A Twelve Step Guide for Healing From Compulsive Sexual Behavior. Minneapolis, MN: CompCare, 1987.

LeSourd, Sandra Simpson. *The Compulsive Woman: How to Break the Bonds of Addiction to Food, Television, Sex, Men, Exercise, Shopping, Alcohol, Drugs, Nicotine, and Much More.* Old Tappan, NJ: Fleming H. Revell, 1987.

Peluso, Emanuel and Lucy. *Women and Drugs: Getting Hooked, Getting Clean.* Minneapolis, MN: CompCare, 1988.

Perlmutter, Judy. *Kick It: Stop Smoking in Five Days.* Tucson, AZ: HP Books, 1986.

ADOPTION

Krementz, Jill. *How It Feels to Be Adopted.* New York: Alfred A. Knopf, 1982.

Lindsay, Jeanne Warren. *Open Adoption: A Caring Option.* Buena Park, CA: Morning Glory, 1987.

———. *Parents, Pregnant Teens, and the Adoption Option: Help for Families.* Buena Park, CA: Morning Glory, 1989.

———. *Pregnant Too Soon: Adoption Is An Option*, rev. ed. Buena Park, CA: Morning Glory, 1988.

AFTER ABORTION COUNSEL

Mannion, Michael T. *Abortion and Healing: A Cry to Be Whole.* Kansas City, MO: Sheed and Ward, 1986.

Michels, Nancy. *Helping Women Recover From Abortion: How to Deal With the Guilt, the Emotional Pain, and the Emptiness.* Minneapolis, MO: Bethany, 1988.

BIRTH CONTROL AND NATURAL FAMILY PLANNING

Clubb, Elizabeth and Jane Knight. *A Comprehensive Guide to Natural Family Planning.* New York: Sterling, 1988.

Silber, Sherman J., M.D. *How Not to Get Pregnant: Your Guide to Simple, Reliable Contraception.* New York: Charles Scribner's, 1987.

CAREER AND EDUCATION

Bramlett, James. *Finding Work: A Handbook.* Grand Rapids, MI: Zondervan, 1986.

Cardozo, Arlene Rossen. *Sequencing: Having It All, But Not All at Once . . . A New Solution for Women Who Want Marriage, Career, and Family.* New York: Atheneum, 1986.

Davidson, Christine. *Staying Home Instead: How to Quit the Working-Mom Rat Race and Survive Financially.* Lexington, MA: D.C. Heath, 1986.

Dreskin, William and Wendy. *The Day Care Decision: What's Best for You and Your Child.* New York: M. Evans & Company, Inc., 1983.

Half, Robert. *The Robert Half Way to Get Hired in Today's Job Market.* New York: Bantam, 1981.

Lowman, Kaye. *Of Cradles and Careers: A Guide to Reshaping Your Job to Include a Baby in Your Life.* Franklin Park, IL: La Leche League, 1984.

Nivens, Beatrice. *Careers for Women Without College Degrees.* New York: McGraw-Hill, 1988.

Sinetar, Marsha. *Do What You Love; The Money Will Follow: Discovering Your Right Livelihood.* New York: Dell, 1989.

Stanton, Jeanne Deschamps. *Being All Things: How to Be a Wife, Lover, Boss, and Mother (and Still Be Yourself).* New York: Doubleday, 1988.

CHOOSING PROFESSIONALS

Danto, Bruce L. *So You Want to See a Psychiatrist?* Salem, NH: Ayer, 1980.

Maurer, Janet R. *How to Talk to Your Doctor: Getting Beyond the Medical Mystique.* New York: Simon & Schuster, 1986.

McCarthy, Eugene et al. *The Second Opinion Handbook: A Guide for Medical Self-Defense.* New York: Nick Lyons Books, 1987.

Saltman, David A. and George Wilgus, III. *The Layman's Guide to Legal Survival: What You Need to Know Before and After You Hire a Lawyer.* Boston, MA: Bob Adams, 1988.

COMMUNICATION

Augsburger, David. *Caring Enough to Confront: How to Understand and Express Your Deepest Feelings Toward Others.* Ventura, CA: Regal, 1981.

Carnegie, Dale. *How to Win Friends and Influence People.* New York: Simon & Schuster, 1964.

Smalley, Gary and John Trent, Ph.D. *The Language of Love: A Powerful Way to Maximize Insight, Intimacy, and Understanding.* Pomona, CA: Focus on the Family, 1988.

CRISIS MANAGEMENT

Kushner, Harold S. *When Bad Things Happen to Good People.* New York: Avon, 1981.

Spencer, Anita L. *Crises and Growth: Making the Most of Hard Times.* Mahweh, NJ: Paulist, 1988.

Stearns, Ann Kaiser. *Living Through Personal Crisis.* New York: Ballentine, 1987.

DEATH

Kubler-Ross, Elisabeth. *On Death and Dying.* New York: Macmillan, 1969.

Landorf, Joyce. *Mourning Song.* Old Tappan, NJ: Fleming H. Revell, 1974. Woman faces own death.

Little, Deborah Whiting. *Home Care for the Dying: A Reassuring, Comprehensive Guide to Physical and Emotional Care.* Garden City, NY: Doubleday, 1985.

Nye, Miriam Baker. *But I Never Thought He'd Die: Practical Help for Widows.* Louisville, KY: John Knox, 1978.

Quinnett, Paul G. *Suicide: The Forever Decision.* New York: Continuum, 1987.

Schaefer, Dan and Christine Lyons. *How Do We Tell the Children?: A Parents' Guide to Helping Children Understand and Cope When Someone Dies.* New York: Newmarket, 1986.

DIET

Astor, Stephen, M.D. *Hidden Food Allergies.* Garden City Park, NY: Avery, 1988.

Brewer, Gail Sforza and Thomas H. *The Brewer Medical Diet for Normal and High Risk Pregnancy: A Leading Obstetrician's Guide to Every Stage of Pregnancy.* New York: Simon & Schuster, 1983.

Feingold, Ben F. and Helene S. *The Feingold Cookbook for Hyperactive Children.* New York: Random House, 1979.

La Leche League International, Roberta Bishop Johnson, ed. *Whole Foods for the Whole Family.* Franklin Park, IL: La Leche League, 1981. Cookbook.

Longacre, Doris Janzen. *More With Less Cookbook.* Scottdale, PA: Herald, 1976.

EMOTIONAL HEALING

Bradshaw, John. *Healing the Shame That Binds You.* Deerfield Beach, FL: Health Communications, 1988.

Branden, Nathaniel. *How to Raise Your Self Esteem.* New York: Bantam, 1987.

Carter, Les. *Good n' Angry: How to Handle Your Anger Positively.* Grand Rapids, MI: Baker, 1983.

———. Paul Meier, and Frank B. Minirth. *Why Be Lonely?: A Guide to Meaningful Relationships.* Grand Rapids, MI: Baker, 1982.

Cerlin, Chuck. *Cleaning Out Your Mental Closet: Transforming Negative Emotions.* Wheaton, IL: Harold Shaw, 1987.

Dalton, Katharina. *Depression After Childbirth: How to Recognize and Treat Postnatal Illness.* New York: Oxford University Press, 1980.

Minirth, Frank B. and Paul D. Meier. *Happiness Is a Choice: A Manual on the Symptoms, Causes and Cures of Depression.* Grand Rapids, MI: Baker, 1988.

Seamonds, David. *Healing for Damaged Emotions.* Wheaton, IL: Victor, 1987.

Smedes, Lewis B. *Forgive and Forget: Healing the Hurts We Don't Deserve.* New York: Pocket, 1984.

FAMILY LIVING

Briggs, Dorothy Corkill. *Your Child's Self-Esteem: The Key to His Life*. New York: Doubleday, 1975.

Broad, Laura Peabody and Nancy Towner Butterworth. *The Playgroup Handbook*. New York: St. Martin's, 1974. How to start a playgroup.

Clegg, Averil and Anne Woollett. *Twins From Conception to Five Years*. New York: Van Nostrand Reinhold, 1983.

Crook, William G., M.D., and Laura Stevens. *Solving the Puzzle of Your Hard-to-Raise Child*. New York: Random House, 1987.

McCullough, Bonnie Runyan and Susan Walker Monson. *401 Ways to Get Your Kids to Work at Home*. New York: St. Martin's, 1981.

Procaccini, Dr. Joseph and Mark W. Kiefaber. *Parent Burnout*. Garden City, NY: Doubleday, 1983.

Smalley, Gary. *The Key to Your Child's Heart*. Waco, TX: Word, 1984.

Touw, Kathleen. *Parent Tricks-of-the-Trade: 1,280 Hints for Your First Ten Years of Parenting*. Mount Rainer, MD: Gryphon, 1987.

FINANCIAL MANAGEMENT

Blue, Ron. *Master Your Money: A Step-by-Step Plan for Financial Freedom*. Nashville, TN: Thomas Nelson, 1986.

Burkett, Larry. *Answers to Your Family's Financial Questions*. Pomona, CA: Focus on the Family, 1987.

Flanagan, Joan. *Grass Roots Fundraising Book: How to Raise Money in Your Community*. Chicago, IL: Contemporary, 1984.

HEALTH

Bergren, Wendy. "Mom Is Very Sick—Here's How to Help." Pomona, CA: Focus on the Family, 1982. Written by a terminally ill mother.

Feingold Association of the United States. *The Feingold Handbook*. Alexandria, VA: Feingold Association of the United States, 1986. How to determine food or additive sensitivity.

Gaes, Sissy. "My Child Is Very Sick—Here's How to Help." Pomona, CA: Focus on the Family, 1989. To be given to friends.

Harrison, Michael. *The Unborn Patient*, 2nd ed. Philadelphia, PA: W. B. Saunders, 1990. Medical treatment, surgery for the unborn.

Harwell, Amy with Kristina Tomasik. *When Your Friend Gets Cancer: How You Can Help*. Wheaton, IL: Harold Shaw, 1987.

Lewis, Kathleen. *Successful Living With Chronic Illness*. Garden City Park, NY: Avery, 1985.

McIlhaney, Joe S., Jr., M.D. *1250 Health-Care Questions Women Ask*. Grand Rapids, MI: Baker, 1985.

Moffatt, Betty Clare. *When Someone You Love Has AIDS: A Book of Hope for Family and Friends*. New York: Nal Penguin, 1986.

Murphy, Judith K. *Sharing Care: The Christian Ministry of Respite Care*. New York: Pilgrim, 1986.

HUMOR

Bombeck, Erma. *Family: The Ties That Bind . . . and Gag!* New York: Random House, 1988.

Eberhart, Elvin. *In the Presence of Humor: A Guide to the Humorous Life*. New Salem, OR: Pilgrim, 1985.

Meberg, Marilyn. *Choosing the Amusing*. Portland, OR: Multnomah, 1986.

Snyder, Bernadette McCarver. *Dear God, I Have This Terrible Problem: A Housewife's Secret Letters*. Liguori, MO: Liguori, 1983.

Welliver, Dotsy. *Smudgkin Elves and Other Lame Excuses*. Winanakake, IN: Light and Life, 1981.

INFANT CARE

Brazelton, T. Berry. *Infants and Mothers: Differences in Development*, rev. ed. New York: Dell, 1983.

Harrison, Helen. *The Premature Baby Book: A Parents' Guide for Coping and*

Caring in the First Year. New York: St. Martin's, 1983.

Hull, Karen. *The Mommy Book: Advice for New Mothers From Women Who've Been There.* Grand Rapids, MI: Zondervan, 1986.

Krauss, Michael with Sue Castle. *Your New Born Baby: Everything You Need to Know, Featuring Joan Lunden.* New York: Warner, 1988.

La Leche League International. *The Womanly Art of Breastfeeding.* Franklin Park, IL: La Leche League, 1981.

Lindsay, Jeanne Warren. *Teens Parenting.* Buena Park, CA 90620: Morning Glory, 1981.

Sears, William, M.D. *The Fussy Baby: How to Bring Out the Best in Your High Need Child.* Franklin Park, IL: La Leche League, 1985.

Thevenin, Tine. *The Family Bed: An Age-Old Concept in Child Rearing.* Garden City Park, NY: Avery, 1985.

INSPIRATION AND MEDITATION

Brenneman, Helen Good. *Meditations for the Expectant Mother.* Scottdale, PA: Herald, 1968.

———. *Meditations for the New Mother.* Scottdale, PA: Herald, 1953.

Brin, Ruth F. *Harvest: Collected Poems and Prayers.* New York: Reconstructionist, 1986. Jewish poetry.

Casey, Karen and Martha Vanceburg. *The Promise of a New Day: A Book of Daily Meditations.* New York: Harper/Hazleden, 1983.

Fishel, Ruth. *Time for Joy: Daily Affirmations.* Pompano Beach, FL: Health, 1988.

LIFE AND STRESS MANAGEMENT

Braiker, Harriet B., Ph.D. *The Type E Woman: How to Overcome the Stress of Being Everything to Everybody.* New York: Dodd, Mead, 1986.

Bright, Dr. Deborah. *Creative Relaxation: Turning Your Stress Into Positive Energy.* New York: Harcourt Brace Jovanovich, 1979.

Culp, Stephanie. *How to Get Organized When You Don't Have the Time.* Cincinnati, OH: Writer's Digest, 1986.

DeRosis, Helen A. *Women and Anxiety.* New York: Dell, 1981. Twenty-step program to deal with anxiety.

Felton, Sandra. *The Messies Manual: The Procrastinator's Guide to Good Housekeeping.* Old Tappan, NJ: Fleming H. Revell, 1981.

Minirth, Frank et al. *How to Beat Burnout: Help for Men and Women.* Chicago, IL: Moody, 1986.

Whitfield, Charles L., M.D. *Healing the Child Within: Discovery and Recovery for Adult Children of Dysfunctional Families.* Deerfield Beach, FL: Health, 1987.

Woititz, Janet. *Adult Children of Alcoholics.* Pompano Beach, FL: Health, 1983.

LOVE MANAGEMENT

Cowan, Dr. Connell and Dr. Melvyn Kinder. *Smart Women, Foolish Choices: Finding the Right Men/Avoiding the Wrong Ones.* New York: Clarkson N. Potter Signet, 1985.

Gullo, Stephen, Ph.D., and Connie Church. *Loveshock: How to Recover From a Broken Heart and Love Again.* New York: Simon & Schuster, 1988.

Marshall, Sharon. *Surviving Separation and Divorce: How to Keep Going When You Don't Really Want To.* Grand Rapids, MI: Baker, 1988.

Norwood, Robin. *Women Who Love Too Much: When You Keep Wishing and Hoping He'll Change.* Los Angeles, CA: Jeremy P. Taner, 1985.

Schaeffer, Brenda. *Is It Love or Is It Addiction?: Falling Into Healthy Love.* New York: Harper and Row, 1987.

Stafford, Tim. *Worth the Wait: Love, Sex, and Keeping the Dream Alive.* Wheaton, IL: Tyndale, 1988.

MARRIAGE ENRICHMENT

Cirner, Randall and Therese. *10 Weeks to a Better Marriage.* Ann Arbor, MI: Servant, 1985.

Lindsay, Jeanne Warren. *Teenage Marriage: Coping With Reality.* Buena Park, CA: Morning Glory, 1988.

Mylander, Charles. *Running the Red Lights.* Ventura, CA: Regal, 1986. Affairs.

Rainey, Dennis and Barbara. *The Questions Book for Marriage Intimacy.* Phoenix, AZ: Questar, 1988.

Williams, Pat and Jill. *Rekindled.* Old Tappan, NJ: Fleming H. Revell, 1985. Rebuilding a crumbling marriage.

Wright, H. Norman and Wes Roberts. *Before You Remarry: A Guide to Successful Remarriage.* Eugene, OR: Harvest House, 1988.

PERSONAL GROWTH

Briggs, Dorothy Corkille. *Celebrate Yourself: Enhancing Your Own Self-Esteem.* New York: Doubleday, 1986.

Lindquist, Marie. *Holding Back: Why We Hide the Truth About Ourselves.* Center City, MN: Hazelden, 1987.

Seamonds, David A. *Putting Away Childish Things.* Wheaton, IL: Victor, 1982. Maturity.

Wegscheider-Cruse, Sharon. *Learning to Love Yourself: Finding Your Self-Worth.* Deerfield Beach, FL: Health, 1987.

PREGNANCY AND BIRTH

"Bill." *Daddy, I'm Pregnant.* Portland, OR: Multnomah, 1987. Pregnant teen.

Brinkley, Ginny, Linda Goldberg, and Janice Kukar. *Your Child's First Journey: A Guide to Prepared Birth From Pregnancy to Parenthood.* Garden City Park, NY: Avery, 1982.

Childbirth Association of Rochester, Inc. *A Labor of Love: A Guide to Family-Centered Cesarean Birth.* Garden City Park, NY: Avery, 1987.

Girard, Linda Wolvoord. *At Daddy's on Saturdays.* Niles, IL: A. Whitman, 1987. Storybook about a child of divorce.

Heil, Ruth. *My Child Within.* Westchester, IL: Good News, 1983. Journal of pregnancies.

Heiman, Carrie J. *The Nine-Month Miracle: A Journal for the Mother-to-Be.* Ligouri, MO: Ligouri, 1986. Journal to fill in.

Kitzinger, Shelia. Photography by Lennart Nilsson. *Being Born.* New York: Grosset & Dunlap, 1986. Photos of unborn children.

———. *Birth Over Thirty.* New York: Penguin, 1985.

Koch, Janice. *Our Baby: A Birth and Adoption Story.* Chicago, IL: Perspective Press, 1985. Children's book.

Olkin, Sylvia Klein. *Positive Pregnancy Fitness.* Garden City Park, NY: Avery, 1987.

Verny, Thomas, M.D., with John Kelly. *The Secret Life of the Unborn Child.* New York: Dell, 1981. Psychology of the unborn.

PREGNANCY AND INFANT LOSS

Cohen, Marion. *An Ambitious Sort of Grief: Pregnancy and Neo-Natal Loss.* Las Colinas, TX: Liberal Press, 1986. Mother's journal.

Gryte, Marilyn. *No New Baby.* Omaha, NE: Centering Corporation, 1988. Children's picture book.

Ilse, Sherokee. *Empty Arms: Coping With Miscarriage, Stillbirth and Infant Death.* Long Lake, MN: Wintergreen, 1982.

——— and Susan Erling. "Planning a Precious Goodbye After Miscarriage, Stillbirth, or Infant Death." Wayzata, MN: Pregnancy and Infant Loss Center, 1984.

——— and Linda Hammer Burns. "Sibling Grief After Miscarriage, Stillbirth, or Infant Death." Wayzata, MN: Pregnancy and Infant Loss Center, 1984.

Page, Carole Gift. *Misty, Our Momentary Child.* Westchester, IL: Crossway, 1987. Dying baby.

Semchyshyn, Stefan, M.D., and Carol Coleman. *How to Prevent Miscarriage and Other Crises of Pregnancy: A Leading High-Risk Doctor's Prescription for Carrying Your Baby to Term.* New York: Macmillan, 1989.

Webster, Robert. "Letters to Geoffrey: A Father's Letters to His Premature Son From Birth to Death." Omaha, NE: Centering Corporation, 1988.

SINGLE PARENTING

Ashton, Betty. *Betty Ashton's Guide to Living on Your Own for the Very First Time.* Boston, MA: Little, Brown, 1988.

Reed, Bobbie. *I Didn't Plan to Be a Single Parent.* St. Louis, MO: Concordia, 1981.

Swihart, Judith J. and Steven L. Brigham. *Helping Children of Divorce.* Downers Grove, IL: Intervarsity, 1982.

SPECIAL NEEDS CHILD

Anderson, Winifred, Stephen Chitwood, and Deidre Hayden. *Negotiating the Special Education Maze: A Guide for Parents and Teachers.* Kensington, MD: Woodbine House, 1989.

Cunningham, Cliff and Patricia Sloper. *Helping Your Exceptional Baby: A Practical and Honest Approach to Raising a Mentally Handicapped Baby.* New York: Pantheon, 1981.

Duckworth, Marion. *Families of Handicapped Children.* Elgin, IL: David C. Cook, 1988. How a church can help.

Pueschel, Siegfried M. and James C. Bernier. *The Special Child: A Source Book for Parents of Children With Developmental Disabilities.* Baltimore, MD: Paul H. Brooks, 1988.

Schwartz, Sue, Ph.D., and Joan E. Heller Miller. *The Language of Toys: Teaching Communication Skills to Special-Needs Children.* Kensington, MD: Woodbine House, 1988.

Stray-Gunderson, Karen. *Babies With Down Syndrome: A New Parents' Guide.* Kensington, MD: Woodbine House, 1986.

Taylor, John. *The Hyperactive Child and the Family: The Complete What-to-Do Handbook.* New York: Dodd, Mead, 1983.

Thompson, Charlotte E., M.D. *Raising a Handicapped Child.* New York: Ballentine, 1986.

SPIRITUAL GROWTH

Booth, Father Leo. *Meditations for Compulsive People: God in the Odd.* Deerfield Beach, FL: Health, 1987.

Chapian, Marie. *His Thoughts Toward Me.* Minneapolis, MN: Bethany, 1987.

de Champlain, Sister Adrienne. *How to Evangelize Myself, First of All!* Available free from Sister Adrienne at St. Anthony Convent, 122 School Street, Taunton, MA 02780.

Green, Melody. *". . . but I can't forgive myself!"* Lindale, TX: Last Days Ministries, 1985.

Hybels, Bill. *Too Busy Not to Pray: Slowing Down to Be With God.* Downers Grove, IL: InterVarsity, 1988.

Kushner, Harold. *When All You've Ever Wanted Isn't Enough: The Search for Life That Matters.* New York: Simon & Schuster, 1986.

Rosage, David E. *The Lord Is My Shepherd: Praying the Psalms.* Ann Arbor, MI: Servant, 1984.

Sherrer, Quin. *How to Pray for Your Children.* Lynnwood, WA: Aglow, 1986.

Yancy, Philip. *Where Is God When It Hurts?* Grand Rapids, MI: Zondervan, 1977.

Works Consulted

In addition to several books mentioned in Appendix I, the following sources were also used in writing this book.

"Adoption: A Loving Choice." Toronto, Ontario: Life Cycle Books, 1986.

"The Adoption Option: Is It for You?" Minneapolis, MN: Adoption Option Committee, Inc., 1982.

"AIDS Virus Infects Infants, Children With a Deadly Vengeance." Newport, RI: *Newport Daily News* 9 March 1988: A-8.

Allison, Christine. "A Child to Lead Us." *The Human Life Review* xv.3 (Summer 1989): 97-102.

American Academy of Pediatrics and American College of Obstetricians and Gynecologists. "Herpes Simplex Infections." Guidelines for Perinatal Care. Ed. Fredric D. Frigoletto, M.D., and George A. Little, M.D. 2nd ed. Elk Grove Village, IL: American Academy of Pediatrics, 1988. 143-49.

American College of Obstetricians and Gynecologists. Obstetric Anesthesia and Analgesia. ACOG Technical Bulletin 112. Washington, DC: American College of Obstetricians and Gynecologists, January 1988.

Apgar, Virginia, M.D., and Joan Beck. *Is My Baby All Right?* New York, NY: Trident, 1972.

Bachrach, Christine A. and Marjorie C. Horn. "Sexual Activity Among US Women of Reproductive Age." *American Journal of Public Health* March 1988: 320-21.

Banks, Adelle M. "Is Rape Sometimes OK?" Providence, RI: *The Providence Journal* 1 May 1988: A-1, 29.

Barnes, Emilie. *More Hours in My Day*. Eugene, OR: Harvest House, 1982.

Barry, Ellen. "Imprisoned Mothers Face Extra Hardships." *The National Prison Project Journal* 14 (Winter 1987): 1-4.

———. "Quality of Prenatal Care for Incarcerated Women Challenged." *Youth Law News* November-December 1985: 1-4.

Beijian, John R. et al. "In Utero Fetal Surgery," Res. 73 (1-81), Council on Scientific Affairs. *Journal of the American Medical Society* 16 September 1983: 1443-44.

Benson, Herbert. *The Relaxation Response*. New York, NY: William and Morrow, 1975.

Bergel, Gary. *When You Were Formed in Secret*. Elyria, OH: Intercessors for America, 1989.

Berkowitz, Gertrude S. et al. "Delayed Childbearing and the Outcome of Pregnancy." *The New England Journal of Medicine* 8 March 1990: 659-64.

Birch, William G., M.D. "A Doctor Discusses Pregnancy." Chicago, IL: Budlong, 1984.

Boston Women's Health Book Collective. *Our Bodies, Ourselves: A Book By and For Women*. New York, NY: Simon & Schuster, 1973.

Boyle, Charles, ed., et al. *The World Book Illustrated Home Medical Encyclopedia*. Chicago, IL: World-Book, Childcraft International, 1980. 4 vols.

Braham, Regina and Bonnie MacAdams Mele. *Life Without Violence, Life Without Fear: A Handbook for Abused Women.* Morristown, NJ: Jersey Battered Women's Service, Inc., n.d.

Brody, Herb. "The Body in Question: How to Stay Healthy at the PC." *PC/ Computing* March 1989: 140-144.

Brody, Jane E. *How a Mother Affects Her Unborn Baby.* Bethesda, MD: National Institute of Child Health and Human Development. Reprinted from Woman's Day Magazine, 1970.

———. "When One Just Doesn't Seem to Satisfy." Providence, RI: *The Providence Sunday Journal* 5 June 1988: E-3.

Canadian Catholic Conference. *The First Days of Human Life.* Ottawa, Ontario, Canada: CCC Publications Service, 1970.

Chesley, Leon C., Ph.D. "The Remote Prognosis for Pregnant Women With Rheumatic Heart Disease." *American Journal of Obstetrics and Gynecology* 1 March 1968: 732-42.

"The Classroom Womb." Los Angeles, CA: *Living World* 1.4 (Summer, 1986): 28.

Cohen, Marion. *She Was Born, She Died.* Omaha, NE: Centering Corporation, 1983.

Counseling and Research Department of Warnke Ministries. "The Philosophy and Practice of Satanism." Danville, KY: Warnke Ministries, September 1987.

Cowart, Virginia. "First-Trimester Prenatal Diagnostic Method Becoming Available in U.S." *Journal of the American Medical Association* 9 September 1983: 1249-50.

Critelli, Ida and Tom Schick. *Unmarried and Pregnant: What Now?* Toronto, Ontario: Life Cycle, 1977.

Crooks, Cheryl. "Healing the Unborn." *Parents* June 1988: 138-43.

Dabilis, Andrew J. and Richard Knox. "Random Tests Show AIDS Virus in Some Babies." Boston, MA: *The Boston Globe* 27 February 1987: 19, 22.

Davidowitz, Esther. "What Experienced Mothers Say." *The Catholic Digest* March 1988: 83-85.

"D.C.'s Teen Mothers Bring Their Babies to School." Providence, RI: *The Providence Sunday Journal* 8 January 1989: B-10. Reprinted from *The Washington Post.*

DeLyser, Femmy. *Jane Fonda's Workout Book for Pregnancy, Birth, and Recovery.* New York, NY: Simon & Schuster, 1982.

Dobson, James C. *Parenting Isn't for Cowards.* Waco, TX: Word, 1987.

Doyle, Larry. "Preemies Get Head Start on Normalcy." Newport, RI: *Newport Daily News* 21 July 1987: 10.

Doyle, Rosaleen. "Relating to the Severely Retarded Person: A Nurse's View." Fairfax, VA: *The National Pro-Life Journal* 7.2 (Spring 1982): 14-16.

Elliott, John. "Abortion for 'Wrong' Sex: An Ethical-Legal Dilemma." *Journal of the American Medical Association* 5 October 1979: 1455-56.

Erling, Susan, ed., et al. "Loss and the Couple." *Loving Arms* November 1987. Wayzata, MN: Pregnancy and Infant Loss Center.

———. "Self-Care and the Griever." *Loving Arms* February 1988. Wayzata, MN: Pregnancy and Infant Loss Center.

Ervin, Paula. *Women Exploited: The Other Victims of Abortion.* Huntington, IN: Our Sunday Visitor, 1985.

Esper, George. "The Children of AIDS." Newport, RI: *The Newport Daily News* 31 August 1988: A-9.

Exercise Before and After Childbirth. Los Angeles, CA: Ross Laboratories, 1985.

Family and Corrections Network News. Waynesboro, VA: Family and Corrections Network 1.1 (August-September 1988): 5, 8, 9.

Festa, Susan. "Coming Back After Pregnancy." *Women's Sports and Fitness* April 1987: 32.

"Fetal Alcohol Advisory Debated." *Science* 6 November 1981: 642-45.

Finegan, Jo-Anne K. et al. "Child Outcome Following Mid-Trimester Amniocentesis: Development, Behaviour, and Physical Status at Age Four Years." *British Journal of Obstetrics and Gynecology.* January 1990: 32-40.

—— et al. "Infant Outcome Following Mid-Trimester Amniocentesis: Development and Physical Status at Age Six Months." *British Journal of Obstetrics and Gynecology.* October 1985: 1015-23.

—— et al. "Midtrimester Amniocentesis: Obstetric Outcome and Neonatal Neurobehavorial Status." *American Journal of Obstetrics and Gynecology.* 15 December 1984: 989-97.

Finley, Mitch. "Large Families." *National Catholic Register* 29 July 1986: 1, 10.

Freudenheim, Milt. "Scientific Advances and Savings Spur a Growing Home Health Care Business." Providence, RI: *The Providence Journal* (Reprinted from *The New York Times*) 15 May 1988: F-8.

Fried, Peter A. and Harry Oxorn. *Smoking for Two: Cigarettes and Pregnancy.* New York, NY: The Free Press (MacMillan), 1980.

Friedman, Rochelle, M.D., and Bonnie Gradstein. *Surviving Pregnancy Loss.* Boston, MA: Little, Brown, 1982.

Fuller, Brian. "Alcohol Can Cause Defects in Unborn." Newport, RI: *Newport Daily News* 29 January 1988: B-6.

Gallup, George, Jr., and Sarah Jones. *One Hundred Questions and Answers: Religion in America.* Princeton, NJ: Princeton Religion Research Center, 1989: 4.

Gaspar, JoAnn. Quoted in "Fatima High Students Lead Nationwide Pro-Life Supporters in March for Life" by Gisele L. Lefebvre. Providence, RI: *The Providence Visitor* 28 January 1988: 15.

"Genetic Omen: Link of 'Fragile X Chromosome' to Mental Impairment Heightens Abortion Issue" and "A Fragile X Surprise: Men Can Pass It On But Not Be Affected." *Wall Street Journal* 18 November 1986: 1, 27.

Genska, Depaul. Letter to author on Genska's work with prostitutes. 11 August 1986.

Goldhaber, Marilyn K. et al. "The Risk of Miscarriage and Birth Defects Among Women Who Use Visual Display Terminals During Pregnancy." *American Journal of Industrial Medicine* 13 (1988): 695-706.

Grieving. Spec. issue of *Intensive Caring Unlimited* Quakertown, PA: ICU-FAMLEE 4.6 (November/December 1986).

Grisez, Germain. *Abortion: The Myths, the Realities, and the Arguments.* New York, NY: Corpus, 1970.

Grover, John W., M.D. *VD—The ABC's.* Englewood Cliffs, NJ: Prentice-Hall, 1972.

Guarino, Jean. "Women Who've Had Abortions." *Catholic Twin Circle* 10 March 1985: 5, 8, 9.

Haddow, James E., M.D., and James N. Macri, Ph.D. "Prenatal Screening for Neural Tube Defects." *Journal of the American Medical Association* 10 August 1979: 515-16.

Handley, Robert with Pauline Neff. *Anxiety and Panic Attacks: Their Cause and Cure.* New York, NY: Rawson, 1985.

Harris, Jean. *"They Always Call Us Ladies": Stories From Prison.* New York, NY: Charles Scribner's, 1988.

Hecht, Frederick et al. "Caution About Chorionic Villi Sampling in the First Trimester." *The New England Journal of Medicine* 24 May 1984.

Henry, Debra. "Meet the Abortion Providers." Chicago, IL: Pro-Life Action League, n.d.

Houck, Catherine. "How to Beat a Bad Mood." *Reader's Digest* January 1989: 93-95.

Ilse, Sherokee. "How Do I Tell the Children?" *Loving Arms* February 1987: 3. Wayzata, MN: Pregnancy and Infant Loss Center.

—— and Susan Erling. *What Next? After Miscarriage, Stillbirth, or Infant Death.* Wayzata, MN: Pregnancy and Infant Loss Center, 1984.

"Infant With New Heart Progressing Well." Providence, RI: *The Providence Sunday Journal* 21 December 1986: A-10.

Jarema, William. "Exercise, Laughter, Prayer Can Be Remedies for Stress." Providence, RI: *The Providence Visitor* 11 May 1989: 30.

Johnson, Dr. S. Marvin and Joy et al. "Death of an Infant Twin." *Intensive Caring Unlimited*, Quakertown, PA: ICU-FAMLEE 3.6 (November/December

1985): 1, 9, 11. Reprinted from *Death of an Infant Twin*. Omaha, NE: Centering Corp.

Kolata, Gina. "Panel Urges Newborn Sickle Cell Screening." *Science* 17 April 1987: 259-60.

Koop, C. Everett, M.D. "The Surgeon General's Report on Acquired Immune Deficiency Syndrome." Washington, DC: U.S. Department of Health and Human Services, n.d.

Kort, Michele. "Can Maternity Make You a Better Athlete?" *Women's Sports and Fitness* May 1986: 38-40, 58.

Langston, Dr. Deborah P. *Living With Herpes*. Garden City, NY: Doubleday, 1983.

Leboyer, Frederick. *Birth Without Violence*. New York, NY: Alfred A. Knopf, 1975.

Legrand-Hosale, C. et al. "If Parents Were Hired, Would You Apply?" Milwaukee, WI: Greater Milwaukee Committee for Unmarried Parent Services, 1986.

Levesque, Dorothy J. "Coping With Stress: Difficult But Possible." Providence, RI: *The Providence Visitor* 11 February 1988: 24.

Lewis, Howard R. and Martha E. *The Parent's Guide to Teenage Sex and Pregnancy*. New York, NY: St. Martin's, 1980.

"Life Before Birth." Westchester, IL: Good News, 1985.

Linn, Matthew et al. *At Peace With the Unborn: A Book for Healing*. Mahwah, NJ: Paulist, 1985.

Lowe, Sarah Fisher. "Single Military Moms Spark Changes in System." Newport, RI: *The Newport Daily News* 23 July 1986: 5.

Macfarlane, Aidan. *The Psychology of Childbirth*. Cambridge, MA: Harvard University Press, 1977.

Maloof, George E., M.D. "The Consequences of Incest: Giving and Taking Life." *The Psychological Aspects of Abortion*. Ed. David Mall and Walter Watts, M.D. Washington, DC: University Publications of America, 1979: 73-101.

Marecek, Mary. *Say "No!" to Violence: Voices of Women Who Experience Violence*. Somerville, NJ: Respond, Inc., 1983.

Marwick, Charles. "Controversy Surrounds Use of Test for Open Spina Bifida." *Journal of the American Medical Association* 5 August 1983: 575-77.

McGuire, Paula. *It Won't Happen to Me: Teenagers Talk About Pregnancy*. New York, NY: Delacourt, 1983.

"A Medical Milestone: Surgery Before Birth." Providence, RI: *The Providence Journal*, East Bay Ed. 8 October 1986: A-1, 2. Reprinted from *The New York Times*.

"Milestones of Early Life." Taylor, AZ: Heritage House, 1985.

"Miracle Baby Celebrates Second Birthday." Washington, DC: *National Right to Life News* 21 August 1986: 4.

Morring, Frank, Jr. "Armed Forces Addresses Pregnancy." Providence, RI: *The Providence Journal-Bulletin* 24 August 1986: B-2.

Morris, Heather, M.D., and Lorraine Williams. "Physical Complications of Abortion." Research Reports 2. Toronto, Ontario: Human Life Research Institute, 1985.

"Mystery Surrounds Coma Pregnancies." Providence, RI: *The Providence Journal* 5 March 1989: B-3.

Nathanson, Bernard M., M.D. New York, NY: *Bernadell Technical Bulletin* 2.1 (January 1990): 4-5.

"New Schools Accommodating the Handicapped." Providence, RI: *The Providence Journal* 5 February 1989: B-7. Reprinted from *The New York Times*.

New York University Medical Center. "Baby Blues: New Mom's Reaction Can Be Serious." Newport, RI: *The Newport Daily News* 4 March 1989: B-8.

Oettinger, Kathleen B. with Elizabeth C. Mooney. *Not My Daughter: Facing Up to Adolescent Pregnancy*. Englewood Cliffs, NJ: Prentice-Hall, 1979.

Oggs, Allan C. with Sherry Andrews. *You Gotta Have the Want To*. Waco, TX: Word, 1987.

Ott, John Nash. "Color and Light: Their Effects on Plants, Animals, and People." Tacoma, WA: *International Journal of Biosocial Research*, Special Subject Issue 7,

1985: 21-26; 8, 1986: 45-49; 12, 1990: 182-185.

Parthun, Mary. "The Psychological Effects of Induced Abortion." Research Reports 2. Toronto, Ontario: Human Life Research Institute, 1985.

Pearson, Jack W., M.D. "The Management of High-Risk Pregnancy." *Journal of the American Medical Association* 9 September 1974: 1439-40.

Pekkanen, John. "The Mounting Toll of Lyme Disease." *Reader's Digest* April 1989: 91-92.

Pepper, Margaret. *The Harper Religious and Inspirational Quotation Companion.* New York, NY: Harper & Row, 1989.

Policy Recommendations on Families of Adult Offenders: Proceedings of the First National Leadership Conference on Families of Adult Offenders. Waynesboro, VA: Family and Corrections Network, 1986.

Powledge, Tabitha M. and John Fletcher. "Guidelines for the Ethical, Social and Legal Issues in Prenatal Diagnosis: A Report From the Genetics Research Group of the Hastings Center, Institute of Society, Ethics and Life Sciences." *The New England Journal of Medicine*, 300 (1979): 168-172.

"Pre-Birth Surgery Saves Baby." *Right to Life Educational Foundation Bulletin.* Cincinnati, OH: Right to Life Educational Foundation, Inc., June-July 1986: 3. Reprinted from an article by C. Caras, *Deseret News*, Provo, UT 11 May 1986.

"Pregnant Too Soon?: Facing Teenage Pregnancy." Weymouth, MA: Life Skills Education, 1985.

Prenatal and Postnatal Care. Wilmington, DE: Stuart Pharmaceuticals, n.d.

"Pro-Life Denominational Groups." Pomona, CA: Focus on the Family, Informational Brochure, 1989.

Public Health Information Sheets: "Congenital Heart Defects," "Down Syndrome," "Rh Disease," "Rubella," "Tay-Sachs," "Thalassemia." White Plains, NY: March of Dimes Birth Defects Foundation, n.d.

Pyle, Amy. "Pregnant Inmates Sue Kern County." Fresno, CA: *The Fresno Bee* 9 September 1987: B-5.

"Questions and Answers About the AFP Test." Prenatal Alpha-fetoprotein testing program, Women and Infants Hospital, Providence, RI, n.d.

Rayburn, William F. and Frederick P. Zuspan. *Drug Therapy in Obstetrics and Gynecology.* 2nd ed. Norwalk, CT: Appleton-Century-Crofts, 1986.

Renshaw, Domeena C. "Incest." *Sexual Medicine Today* February 1983: 7-11.

Riggs, Doug. "Cocaine Symptoms Soar in R.I. Births." Providence, RI: *The Providence Sunday Journal* 8 January 1989: A-1, 16.

Rodale Press Editors, compiled by Joanne Mayer. *Be a Healthy Mother, Have a Healthy Baby.* Emmaus, PA: Rodale, 1973.

Roggow, Linda and Carolyn Owens. *Handbook for Pregnant Teenagers.* Grand Rapids, MI: Zondervan, 1985.

Ross, Randy. "VDTs: Are They Safe?" *PC/ Computing* March 1989: 146-47.

Salmon, Jacqui. "From Here to Maternity." *Women's Sports* July 1983: 44-48.

Saltenberger, Ann. *Every Woman Has a Right to Know the Dangers of Legal Abortion.* Glassboro, NJ: Air-Plus Enterprises, 1982.

Saltus, Richard. "Fetal Test Soon Could Be Routine." Boston, MA: *The Boston Globe* 29 July 1985: 33.

Scher, Jonathan and Carol Dix. *Will My Baby Be Normal?* New York, NY: Dial, 1983.

Schwarz, Ted and Duane Empey. *Satanism: Is Your Family Safe?* Grand Rapids, MI: Zondervan, 1988.

Selwyn, Amy. *Genetic Counseling.* White Plains, NY: The National Foundation/ March of Dimes, n.d.

Shaevitz, Marjorie Hansen. *The Superwoman Syndrome.* New York, NY: Warner, 1984.

"Significant Events in a New Life." Taylor, AZ: Heritage House '76, n.d.

Skeat, Walter W. *A Concise Etymological Dictionary of the English Language.* New York, NY: Capricorn, 1963.

Slattery, Helen and Lorraine Williams. *Help—I Need Hope.* Toronto, Ontario: Life Cycle Books, 1983.

Solomon, Dr. Neil. "Medical Mailbag." Newport, RI: *Newport Daily News* 9 May 1986: 22; 16 August 1986: 11.

Stack, Jack M., M.D. "The Father." *Loving Arms* 8.2 (Summer 1989): 5. Wayzata, MN: Pregnancy and Infant Loss Center.

State Department of Agriculture's Human Nutrition Information Service, Home and Garden Bulletin Number 232-1, n.d.

Staying Fit During Pregnancy. San Juan, Puerto Rico: Searle and Company, 1980.

Stein, Loren and Veronique Mistiaen. "Mothers Behind Bars." Boston, MA: *Boston Sunday Herald Magazine* 30 October 1988: 5-8, 16-17.

———. "Pregnant in Prison." *The Progressive* February 1988: 18-21.

Stevenson, Burton. *The Home Book of Quotations: Classical and Modern.* New York, NY: Dodd, Mead & Company, 1935.

"Study and Learning in the Womb." *Science Magazine* 20 July 1984: 302-303.

"Sudden Infant Death Linked to Smoking." Providence, RI: *Providence Sunday Journal* 25 February 1990: D-3.

Suffolk, NY. Introductory Res. No. 1173-88. "A Local Law Providing Employee Protection Against Video Display Terminals." 1 March 1988.

Teenaged and Pregnant: A Time to Stay Healthy. Columbus, OH: Ross Laboratories, 1986.

Thomas, Ellen Lamar with Ellen Postlewaite. "How to Die." *Catholic Digest* March 1988: 110-114.

United States Environmental Protection Agency. "EPA Probe Likely to Identify Electricity as Major New Cancer Risk." Inside EPA Weekly Report, 23 March 1990: 1,6.

Van Buren, Abigail. "Best Care for the Retarded May Not Be in the Home." "Dear Abby." Newport, RI: *Newport Daily News* 9 January 1989: B-10.

Vandagaer, Paula. "Rape and the Pro-Life Pregnancy Service Response." *Heartbeat,* Spring 1984: 4-6.

Vibrant. "One Woman's Story." *Genesis House Newsnotes.* Chicago, IL: Genesis House, Spring. 1989: 2.

Walker, Lenore E. *The Battered Woman.* New York, NY: Harper & Row, 1979.

Walling, Regis. *When Pregnancy Is a Problem.* St. Meinrad, IN: Abbey, 1980.

Wallis, Claudia. "Children Having Children." *Time Magazine* 9 December 1985: 78-90.

"What You Should Know About Hemophilia." Providence, RI: Rhode Island Hemophilia Foundation, n.d.

Williams, Phyllis. *Nourishing Your Unborn Child.* Los Angeles, CA: Nash, 1974.

Willke, Dr. and Mrs. J. C. *Abortion: Questions and Answers.* Cincinnati, OH: Hayes, 1985, rev. 1988.

———. "AIDS and Abortion." Washington, DC: *National Right to Life News* 16 July 1987: 3.

———. "Assault Rape, and Pregnancy (Part III)." Washington, DC: *National Right to Life News* 9 October 1986: 3.

———. "Now: Simple Way to Detect Fetal Heartbeat at Six Weeks." Washington, DC: *National Right to Life News* 3 December 1987: 3.

———. "Viability Under Twenty-Four Weeks." Washington, DC: *National Right to Life News* 11 May 1989: 3, 10.

World-Wide Directory of Pro-Life Emergency Pregnancy Services. White Plains, NY: Alternatives to Abortion, Int., 1988/89.

Worthington-Roberts, Bonnie, Ph.D., and Lynda E. Taylor. *Nutrition During Pregnancy and Breastfeeding.* Chicago, IL: Budlong, 1984.

Young, Carol. "How the Social Worker Can Help Bereaved Parents." *Intensive Caring Unlimited* 3.6 (November/December 1985): 3. Quakertown, PA: ICU-FAM-LEE.

Zimmerman, Martha. *Should I Keep My Baby?* Minneapolis, MN: Bethany, 1983.

Index